Fragile

Fragile

BEAUTY IN CHAOS,
GRACE IN TRAGEDY,
AND THE HOPE THAT
LIVES IN BETWEEN

SHANNON SOVNDAL, M.D.

Published by Gyrfalcon Press, Denver, Colorado
www.shannonsovndal.com

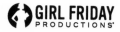

Edited and Designed by Girl Friday Productions
www.girlfridayproductions.com
Editorial: Clete Smith, Ben Grossblatt, Karla Anderson
Interior Design: Paul Barrett
Cover Design: Alban Fischer
Cover and interior photography © 2020 Mike Thurk

ISBN (Paperback): 978-1-7344251-0-9
e-ISBN: 978-1-7344251-1-6
LCCN: 2020900280

First Edition

Printed in the United States of America

To Steph

CONTENTS

AUTHOR'S NOTE

Each chapter is associated with a song in my mind. It could be a lyric, a feeling, or just a connection between the writing and the music. I had originally included quotes from songs at the beginning of each chapter but realized the copyright lawyers would have a field day with me. So, instead, at the beginning of each chapter, I've included the song title and artist. My hope is that you check out some of the music as you make your way through the book.

Sometimes even to live is an act of courage.
Seneca

PROLOGUE

ZEBRA

"Lunatic Fringe" Red Rider

I remember standing motionless in the doctors' lounge, staring at my hands. Things had changed. I was someone different, someone my family and friends might not recognize if I let them in, really let them see my true soul. But that wasn't possible. Not for me. I was too guarded, always guarded, always in control. It wasn't just today that had changed me. It had been everything.

All I wanted to do was see my boys. I wanted proof that they were safe at home; I wanted to see them alive and well, laughing and playing—finding joy in the little things like Legos, action figures, and our dog, Ryder. Instead I was alone, feeling the frantic drone of a busy emergency department. There was no time for reflection or emotion; patients were waiting to be seen. Trauma Room 11 had just given me a cold taste of reality. No superhero saves or knights in shining armor—just the simple fact that sometimes really bad things happen.

In the background, the TV mounted in the corner of the room played ESPN baseball highlights. With the excitement of a lottery winner, the well-groomed commentator extolled the virtues of Alex Rodriguez because he had hit yet another home run. He makes close to $58,000 every time he steps to the plate. I guess he deserves it, the pressure and all. I didn't take note of who won the game, I can only recall Alex.

I stood like a zombie in the middle of the lounge, numb, like the poor zebra you see on Animal Planet after having one of its legs chomped off by a hidden crocodile during a compulsory river crossing in Tanzania. The look, that look, on the zebra's face always struck me as a bit misplaced, because it was devoid of any apparent emotion or concern. Moments from death, tripodding on the far shore, the zebra appeared totally detached and dissociated from its dire predicament. As I stood there, I felt the same as that zebra, vacant of any emotional content. I understood the look. I shouldn't have been able to push my emotions aside, not if I possessed some small fleck of compassion or empathy. Because this wasn't normal. This wasn't what people experienced day to day. At least not normal people.

But I had been trained to be this way. No panic, just a calm journeyman's approach to any affliction, like a mathematician working an equation. Years of preparation, acquiring a skill set, building up my vault, had readied me to stand in the lounge like a zebra.

And so, I stared at my hands to see if I was actually here, to see who I was. Maybe I was hoping to see something different. Anything, really. A tremble, a shake. But I saw nothing. Just my hands. Steady. Solid. Quiet.

The clock clicked, 8:21. It was one of those old-school clocks, like you'd see on the wall back in grade school. I had zoned out looking at a similar clock at my son's last parent-teacher conference. The second hand was rigid and jerky, making a big move forward, then a small move back. Big forward, small back.

Everything fits together, like the pieces of a giant puzzle. The picture becomes clear only when the dark colors blend with the bright. The picture is revealed because of the unity of pieces. I felt the seconds ticking, moving forward from 8:21. Even though it didn't look like it, deep down, the last thirty minutes had kicked my ass. From the outside I was calm, but somewhere inside, the hideous reality of death and suffering screamed and rattled in my well-guarded cage.

PART I

FUNERALS SUCK

"I Grieve" Peter Gabriel

Yeah, funerals suck. I don't know what you want me to say.

BAT PHONE

"Superstition" Stevie Wonder

I had started one of my typical weekend shifts in the ER. I took over the lingering patients from the night doc, caught up with some of the oncoming nurses, and then, trying to ease into the fact that I had to work on Sunday, headed to the cafeteria. I stood in front of the assorted donut tray trying to decide between two favorites—jelly or apple fritter. The jelly is just so overwhelmingly sweet, it could have been a good choice for Sunday. But the sheer volume of the apple fritter was undeniable. As I am a donut connoisseur, the decision was clear.

Apple fritter sitting precariously on a small Styrofoam plate, I grabbed a coffee and headed back toward the ER. The lights overhead passed in rhythm. The speckled linoleum floor, typical in a hospital, glistened underfoot thanks to the overnight polish.

Without spilling or dropping my breakfast, I managed to maneuver my name badge over the silver automatic doorplate and took up my typical position at the chart rack. I indulged in my first bite, and any sense of embarrassment from holding such an obscenely large donut quickly passed.

The patient board looked good: a couple of drunks left over from the night before, one psychotic patient, and a belly pain. For a post-Saturday-night shift, I couldn't complain. If it stayed this way, I figured I'd be able to catch bits of the 49ers game on TV.

Our ER looks pretty standard—old, run-down, and artificially lit. Repeated face-lifts failed to remedy what it really needed: an extreme makeover.

Working in our department feels like sitting on an old tattered couch from your parents' house. It's comfortable, fits your butt nicely, but man, it looks gnarly. If I didn't have such a familiarity with it, I'd probably never think to even sit in it.

ERs might appear cool and high-tech on TV, but in the real world, they usually lack funding and are at least five years behind expected patient volume. Hence, patients are always pissed off because of the long wait, overwhelmed service, and lackluster amenities. Did you know that if an ER has public Wi-Fi, the doctor's rating magically increases? True story. Same if I wear a white coat. But I hate white coats, so I'll take the hit.

If hospital administrators spend money, they usually go for a slick cancer center or some similar high-profile project. Congressmen and journalists like medical facilities that, to steal a term from my marketing friends, "pop." *The Prescott Cancer Center* or *the Kandel Institute of Neuroscience* sounds so much better than *ER renovation*.

As you might guess, emergency departments don't generate large amounts of income for the hospital.

Considering the lack of selection bias for ER patients with a means to pay their bill, the accounting books rarely look good. We treat anyone who walks through the door, rich or poor, young or old, annoying or nice. While our open-door policy allows me to practice what I consider a pure form of medicine, it nevertheless places a financial strain on the system. Bottom line, it's understandable why administrators aren't throwing money our way.

Our ER forms a giant U with a couple of extra straggly limbs. The common work area sits at the center of the U, with patient rooms fanned out on the perimeter. The common work area contains the charge nurses' and ER techs' desks. They sit side by side, facing the same direction, with a slim walkway in between. On the far wall, facing both desks, a large, mounted plasma screen serves as the patient board. It displays pertinent information: name, bed number, arrival time, chief complaint, and pending evaluation studies. In the center of the work area, a long, four-foot-high, wooden cubbyhole structure houses all the charts.

The whole setup reminds me a bit of old-school *Star Trek*. I've found that, although it's not its intended function, the chart rack makes a perfect seat, or captain's chair. When I hop up, I feel like Captain Kirk controlling the entire *Starship Enterprise*. Sitting atop the rack, I have a great view of everything vital in the ER. The patient board lies dead ahead. To the left, I can see the area-wide ER tracker to aid in mass casualty events and county-wide patient flow. To the right, the patient monitors chirp out their regular updates. I also have a good view of the ambulance bay door and am within earshot of the medic "bat phone." Everything an ER doc needs to keep the ER running smoothly. Donut in hand, I prepared for whatever the shift might bring.

As I dipped the fritter in my coffee, I started to banter with some of the staff. "Hey Bruce, where's the flood? Been playing in the sewer again?" Bruce was one of my favorite nurses, and due to his six-foot-three, 260-pound build, his pants always seemed to be an inch too short.

He looked back at me and quipped in his Jersey accent, "Yeah, I was down there with your mom." As I prepared some disparaging remark, the paramedic tone box, a small speaker that sits on the ER techs' desk, interrupted my comeback.

"Community, ahhh, this is Medic 3. We're ... we're five minutes out. We have a three-year-old male." Pause. "CPR in progress."

Not the most informative ring-down, but I imagined the medic had his hands full. I knew him well. The other night we talked about making skateboards and the finer points of woodworking.

Usually laid back, today he sounded distracted and tense. As he talked I could hear the wail of the siren ring out in the background. If you watched this unfold on Thursday night primetime, the Hans Zimmer music would start to build the suspense. But this wasn't TV. This was just a real-world Sunday.

Our tech glanced up at me, depressed the speaker button and replied, "Room 11 on arrival."

Although usually not fazed by much, staff can get a little amped up by a pediatric code. It gets me fired up as well. But in a good way. I actually like sick and critical patients. Like most ER docs, I came out of my training excited to put into practice all that I had learned. The more sick or injured, the better. That might sound a little sick-minded, but that's the truth. That's why I chose this job. Just like firefighters prefer big, nasty fires, ER docs like sick people.

I admit I had a superhero dream. A lot of docs do, even if they don't like to admit it. When things get really bad and people need help, we come to the rescue. That's the dream, straight-up Marvel. But don't judge me. It's a way to make all the sacrifice seem worthwhile. I get to perform all the tasks and skills I painstakingly spent years learning in school, residency, and practice. Every wedding, funeral, or family event I missed—this makes me feel like it was not in vain. This is a moment to make it all justifiable.

I like to break things down to their simplest terms, including patients in the ER. There are three basic types: 1) those who will live regardless of my intervention, 2) those who will die regardless of my intervention, and 3) those who will live or die depending on how well I do my job. I mentally geared up for number three.

Often, when we get a ring-down for an elderly patient in cardiac arrest, the staff positions a body bag on top of the mattress before the patient's arrival, because unlike in Hollywood resuscitations, our efforts on these patients usually fail. Having the bag pre-positioned saves the staff from the awkward task of trying to move a deceased patient into the bag. For a pediatric "COR" (cardiac arrest), the body bag never comes out before the patient arrives.

Right on schedule, the deep, guttural sound of the ambulance's diesel engine rumbled from the bay. With a familiar bang, the ambulance entrance doors swung open. The paramedics surged through the entrance, revealing a sudden wave of activity, and the looks on their faces confirmed the tension I had heard over the radio. Noah, the medic, peered up from his cardiac monitor, and he looked relieved to see me. Patients are like hot potatoes for paramedics, and Noah couldn't wait to pass this potato.

"What's up, Noah?" I said in a calm tone, trying to defuse some apprehension.

"Mom found the kid down in the living room. Unknown total time, but sounds like less than five minutes." To prevent the need for yelling with all the commotion, I leaned in toward Noah as we moved toward Room 11. I could feel the heat and energy emanating from his body. I glanced back as we were turning the corner and caught a glimpse of the mom walking through the bay doors. She was talking with the registration people, and a firefighter held her arm. She looked a bit like the zebra.

"Let's move him over," I said as I unlatched the lower seatbelt holding the boy on the ambulance pram. Grabbing the bottom of the sheet, three of us slid my new patient onto the gurney.

"The kid's been sick with a URI. Been vomiting too. When we arrived, he had agonal respirations. The monitor showed course V-fib. I shocked him once at thirty with no change. Shocked again at sixty, and the patient showed PEA on the monitor. Sorry, I couldn't get a tube, and . . ." Noah swung his head around as if someone had called his name. Realizing he had only heard the background commotion, he turned back to me and finished his report. "And, sorry, Doc, I couldn't get a line for you."

Great. In other words, we don't have jack, I thought. This meant the kid had no breathing tube and no IV access. And no way for me to help. *This is going to be a bit dodgy.*

My high school soccer coach always used to yell at us, "Practice like you play" and "Be consistent!" Aside from my typing class, soccer practice better prepared me for life than any other high school activity. Regardless of the severity of my patient, I try to stick to the same regimented, methodical approach. It starts with the basic ABCs. Airway. Breathing. Circulation. Usually I complete the assessment quickly and easily—an awake, talking patient generally has a good airway, adequate breathing, and at least some degree of circulation. Painfully obvious, this poor little kid had none of these.

Immediately, the ER staff moved into their familiar and pre-orchestrated roles. The monitor revealed the medic's correct assessment: the patient was in PEA (pulseless electrical activity)—a rhythm incompatible with life and not curable by firing up the defibrillator.

First order of business: airway. I moved to the head of the bed and set up for intubation. "How old is he?" I looked up at the sweating paramedic.

"He's three . . . I think," the response came with a nervous glance to his partner.

I looked at the boy's naked and pale little body. My mind began to process the problem. *Newborn's three kilograms. They double by four months—six kilograms. One year—ten kilograms. Three years—fifteen kilograms.*

Based on the child's size, I grabbed a Miller 2 blade laryngoscope and a 5.0 ET (endotracheal) tube. I recalled one of my pediatric professors from residency saying, "Miller blades are better than Macintosh blades for little ones because their vocal cords lie more anterior than adults' cords."

Gently scissoring his jaw open with the index finger and thumb of my right hand, I carefully slipped the blade into his mouth with my left hand. I took care not to pinch the lips or chip a tooth. I pulled forward and upward—tongue, uvula, posterior pharynx, vallecula, and then, thankfully, vocal cords. That's what I was looking for. I passed the tube without incident. Positive breath sounds, absent stomach noises, misting of the tube, and capnometry change all confirmed I had done it right.

Next up: breathing. I asked the respiratory therapist to bag him as I helped secure the tube. I checked her rate. People get excited with kids and often overbreathe when bagging. His chest cavity rose nicely, and although he had air movement on both sides, rales were present. That's the sound of breathing through a snorkel tube when there's still a little water left over after you surface from a dive. The trachea still appeared midline, and I didn't palpate any abnormalities on his chest wall. All this made pneumothorax less likely. With his breathing secured for now, I addressed his circulation.

CPR was in progress. Staff were swarming around the boy's little body. We continued with compressions until it was time for a rhythm check. I squeezed between the nurse and tech to touch the patient. There's a lot of activity around a patient in cardiac arrest. It is typical for the doctor to stand back a bit to maintain control of the entire room and the resuscitation. But intermittently, we have to bounce in to perform a procedure or examine the patient.

I reached down and palpated his brachial artery with one hand—nothing. Then the carotid with the other—nada. I looked up at Sarah, one of our trauma techs, and said, "Continue CPR, please." It's funny because I really did say *please*. The more stressed I get, the more polite and calm I become. I learned that from Dr. Klofas, one of my attendings at Stanford during training. Sarah and the firefighter had already done their little dance to switch positions. Standing on a small stepstool, Sarah began cardiac compressions.

His mom came through the doors of the resuscitation room, and I looked up from her son. I didn't say anything. But our eyes met. I pressed my lips—not a smile or a frown, just a confirmation that I knew who she was. That she was Mom. Even nonmedical people know what CPR means. I'd have to deal with her in a moment. For now, I had to try to get a better handle on her boy.

We have excellent nurses, and they repeatedly have amazed me by placing IV catheters into the smallest of veins. But, unfortunately in this case, that might have taken too long. "Hey, Sue, would you get the IO kit?" I asked.

"Thanks," I said a moment later as she passed the small box over the patient's bed.

The IO (interosseous) device is a hand drill, but instead of connecting to a metal bit, there is a large-bore, beveled-end needle. The technique is simple: drill the needle through the outer cortex of the bone into the marrow. It is down and dirty. It might sound horrible, but it is fast and reliable. From the marrow, fluid and medications can find their way into the patient's general circulation.

We practiced this procedure on chicken bones during residency, but they don't work too well. Actually, letting on to my age just a bit, when I learned this procedure we didn't have a drill. We had the large-bore needle connected to a round, ball-like handle. We would just punch the needle through the skin and bone, like putting a hole in a leather belt. With the pressure exerted by the ball-and-needle device, the chicken legs would occasionally explode. Residents sometimes stuck themselves when the needle lurched through the splintering bone. This happened to poor Espinoza, my partner, during a training lab.

I palpated the small flat area on the inside aspect of the leg just below the knee. With a minimal amount of force due to the spinning drill head, the needle punched through just as advertised. *Much easier than a chicken bone,* I thought.

As the nurse secured the IO line, I noted that the IV fluid stopped flowing. I disconnected the bag and attached a syringe. Gently applying pressure to the plunger seemed to do the trick. *Now we're in business,* I thought. I could start treating the patient with medications and fluid.

I glanced up at the monitor to see the cardiac rhythm and felt a bead of sweat on my forehead. Internally my mind commented on the stressful situation, as if I were observing it at a distance. I thought of my kids and had a moment of pause. *What if it were my son?* I looked at my patient's lean build and no-hassle buzz cut and couldn't help but make the comparison. The thought momentarily sent a chill down my spine. I looked over at his dazed mom. She was caught up in a whirlwind of disbelief that her son was lying limp and motionless. I could feel the emotion welling up inside me. I took a deep breath and shut it down. I pushed my son out of my head and forced myself to think of the boy as a patient, only a patient. A physiologic problem, an equation. *This isn't my emergency. It is his emergency. I'm fine.*

I focused and re-addressed the monitor. Still PEA. *Why is he in PEA?*

Emergency Medicine: A Comprehensive Study Guide is the emergency physician's bible. Because of the editor's name, we call it "Tintinalli." I've always been a bit amused that it is *only* a "study guide." Tintinalli weighs ten and a half pounds, literally, and "condenses" the subject matter of emergency medicine down to 2,127 pages—a readable and memorizable 2,127 pages. Page 187 addresses PEA and it is *bad news*. You know it's serious when it occurs on page 187 of 2127.

> "PEA is due to a profound metabolic abnormality of the myocardium, rendering it non-contractible. At this time, there is NO CLEARLY BENEFICIAL THERAPY."

Simply put, this boy's heart had stopped pumping. The electrical signal continued to propagate, but the muscle fibers failed to respond. The lack of blood flow rendered him pulseless.

Even if the "bible" says there's no clearly beneficial therapy, I still had to try. I'd take possible benefit or even occasional benefit—anything to turn this around. In a split second my mind searched its stored data on PEA, and I recalled the ACLS (Advanced Cardiac Life Support) algorithm for PEA.

I'm a visual person. I see charts, images, and book pages in my mind, and I quickly scanned down the flow diagram I had memorized, and there it was—epinephrine. It's an endogenous catecholamine that potently stimulates alpha- and beta-adrenergic receptors. Simply put, epinephrine acts like adrenaline—the same stuff released when you try to avoid getting hit by a car. It affects the fight-or-flight response of the sympathetic nervous system. Not only does it clamp down the vascular system, delivering more oxygen and blood to the core and brain, it also can kick-start the heart back into action.

Adults are so much easier to deal with than kids in these life-threatening situations. They all get 1 mg of 1:10,000 epinephrine pushed into their IV. Kids are a different story because everything is based on weight. To complicate things, epinephrine comes in two concentrations: 1:1,000 and 1:10,000. One gram in 1,000 milliliters and 1 gram in 10,000 milliliters, respectively. The mode of delivery (IV, intraosseous, intramuscular, subcutaneous, down the breathing tube) determines the concentration. Since I had the IO line in place, my patient needed the less-concentrated version of 1:10,000 at a dose of 0.01 milligrams per kilogram (mg/kg). Fifteen kg (the boy's estimated weight) times 0.01 mg/kg gives a product of 0.15 mg. Converting to milliliters and considering the concentration, I flushed a total dose of 1.5 ml through the IO catheter.

"And let's just go ahead and give him some sugar. Can you grab some D10?" I made eye contact with the nurse standing by the medication drawer.

A short while after injecting the medication into the boy's body, I looked up at Sarah and said, "Hold CPR." My hand again pushed through the crowd and went to his neck. My gloved finger noted the lack of a carotid pulse. I glanced again at the monitor, and it still showed PEA.

Fuck me.

8:12

"Black Hole Sun" Soundgarden

As I stood over the little boy in Trauma Room 11, I silently ran through the ten possible PEA etiologies: hypovolemia, hypoxia, acidosis, hyperkalemia/hypokalemia, hypothermia, overdose, tamponade, tension pneumothorax, heart attack, and pulmonary embolus. Residency had drilled these into my brain. During one of our monthly educational meetings, our director singled me out to stand and then "pimped," or aggressively questioned, me.

"Shannon!" I think I must have been off in space by the way he barked my name. I hadn't been sleeping much. Nobody had. I whipped my head back in his direction. "You've got a patient that rolls into the ER. He's sixty-seven years old, pulseless with CPR in progress. Here's the EKG." An EKG went up on the overhead. Yes, we still used overheads. I was so freaking tired. The trauma rotation was kicking my ass. Time was kicking my ass. I hadn't slept in two days . . . honestly.

A trauma resident's schedule sucks. You're on call every other day. That means that you spent twenty-four hours in the hospital every other day. The day in between these call days is also spent in the hospital—usually starting around 4:00 a.m. and ending close to 7:00 p.m. Essentially a twenty-four–hour day, followed by a fifteen-hour day, followed by a twenty-four-hour day, followed by a fifteen-hour day, followed by a . . . Well, you get it. During my rotation I had two days off during the month.

The word *call* makes it sound so humane, but unfortunately it's not. As the name seems to imply, you might think that the on-call doctor could just sit at home occasionally fielding phone calls. On the contrary, call means the resident has to stay the night in the hospital. I used the word *stay* rather than *sleep*, because at a large tertiary care trauma center like Stanford, little if any downtime exists. Quite typically, a trauma resident could work forty hours straight, relying only on periodic catnaps to get by. There're new laws about this now. But not back in the day when I had to walk uphill in the snow both ways to work. The new rules were designed to protect the patients and keep everyone safe. Future residents would only be able to work eighty hours a week.

I stood before the faculty and residents, having just finished my most recent call day. *Why do they always call on the postcall guy?* I attempted to gather my wits. In a nearly impossible feat for my condition, I recalled the first five causes of PEA. Number six came after a fair amount of delay.

There was only an "Aaaaaaa," followed by the sound of my breathing. The jeering of my residency-mates only added to the complexity of my remaining task. The education in medical school and residency is like drinking from a fire hose. So much knowledge needs to be crammed into your brain during a limited time. This is combined with the lack of sleep and the obvious workload that comes with taking care of patients.

"Come on, the patient is dying. You need to know this," the director said, keeping up the pressure.

I couldn't remember anything else. I repeated the first six answers more quickly, hoping that saying them again would somehow kick-start the rest of my memory. It didn't. I stared down at the floor. I was failing my imaginary patient.

"OK, Shannon. No problem. You'll just have to explain to your patient's family that you're too tired to remember the reason their father died," my director said, raising his eyebrows and shaking his head slightly.

Finally, a buddy came to my rescue. We called him the Minister. That was short for the Minister of Misinformation. We had affectionately given him this name because he always had something to say, whether he knew what the heck he was talking about or not. Fortunately for me, on this occasion, the Minister dialed in the correct answer. I quickly yielded the floor and ended the moronic feeling of standing in front of everyone, mind blank, having nothing to say. I sat and pressed my palms into my eye sockets. If you are ever lacking sleep, you should try it. It feels phenomenal.

I never missed that answer again, the reasons for PEA. I didn't hesitate today with this little boy. Of the ten possible causes, the first two—hypovolemia and hypoxia—seemed the most likely. I checked to see that the fluid was still flowing. It was. The ventilator had the proper parameters set.

As I walked around the gurney to the other side, I cut between the boy and his mother. I wanted to believe that she still felt numb, but at that moment I could see, I could feel, that she didn't. Soul to soul, mother to son. Life was flowing away from him, vaporizing into oblivion.

I didn't intend to, but I caught a glimpse of her face, only briefly. It was terrible. *Horrific* is a better word. I saw her swollen, tear-filled eyes, deep and dark. Her black hair was smeared against her forehead, clumped and moist from her sweat and tears. She had the look of a character in *Game of Thrones*. If you don't watch it, there is something you should know: everyone dies. I mean everyone.

Her face contorted for a moment, Guantanamo Bay torture style.

My entire body felt heavy, like my arms and legs were filled with metal pellets. It wasn't from physical fatigue; it was from pure emotional suck. It was from watching someone die. Watching my patient die. My kid die.

I focused on the boy's face and paused. He looked tired too. His cheeks pulled inward, and the bony structure of his face was *too* notable. Healthy kids have chubby cheeks and full skin. He had the opposite. It already looked like he was becoming a skeleton. His eyes were open, but they focused on nothing. Dark and sunken into his skull.

I scanned down his body again, looking for any clues. His physique showed his previous health. His body looked fit and toned, his chest and abdominal muscles primed from hours of rolling around on the floor playing ninja and superhero. Unfortunately, he wasn't a superhero. Unfortunately, I wasn't a superhero.

I moved from between the boy and his mom, awkwardly but purposefully. She was sitting in a chair off to the patient's right. I gained some relief from the vortex of being in that space. I again caught her in my peripheral vision. I wasn't man enough to look straight at her. Her veins were bulging and her facial muscles were taut, but her expression seemed void. The tension of a thousand lifetimes lost pulled at my soul. I tensed in fear. It was trying to consume me. I focused again. My training. My breathing. Big forward, small back. I steadied myself by laying one hand on the patient's arm, the other on the pram, and dug all my toes into the soles of my clogs.

Only a moment passed.

I was back. I slid the ultrasound machine over and squirted the cold gel on his white, smooth chest. It magnified the mottled and purplish appearance of his skin. Just yesterday I had grabbed the same bottle to check out a healthy fetus in my pregnant patient. Taking the ultrasound probe, I situated the transducer between the ribs so the sound waves could clearly reflect off the heart.

My eyes darted between the ultrasound's screen and the cardiac monitor. The monitor still showed PEA. On the ultrasound, I made out the four chambers of the heart and the pericardial sac. Not that I expected the finding, but no large volume of fluid had collected between the heart and the pericardium, no cardiac tamponade.

Am I missing something? Breathe in, breathe out. Big forward, small back. *Focus on the moment.* The pictures from my textbooks were visible in crisp definition. My neural network catapulted between symptom and sign, connecting the dots between diagnosis and treatment.

I looked toward the nurse. "Push some of that fluid. Another twenty per kilo." I said it quietly, but like I was a little annoyed. I wasn't annoyed at the nurse, or the patient, or the fluid needing to be pushed. I was annoyed that I was losing. I was annoyed at myself. And at God. I couldn't change the outcome. I checked the clock—8:04. "Work on another line. And swap out compressions." I gave a hand gesture to the firefighter now doing CPR. "We got a temp yet?"

Glancing up to my right, I saw that the green-colored heart tracing on the monitor continued to show PEA.

"He's burning up—103." The nurse informed me of the temperature reading from his Foley catheter.

I heard the familiar pop as the X-ray tech jerked the chest film into place on the light box. I moved close to note the abnormal image, but didn't have to. It looked abnormal from across the room. Way too much white. This is why his lungs had sounded like the water-filled snorkel.

X-rays are all about density. Air is less dense than fluid, which is less dense than bone. Normally, air fills the lungs so the X-ray beams readily pass to the film, turning the image black. However, this poor kid's lungs were filled with junk—bacteria, fluid, inflammatory mediators, and white blood cells—which blocked the radiation from passing to the X-ray plate. A simple pneumonia causes a small area of white on an X-ray. This boy had the Megatron of pneumonia. It was everywhere.

I don't know why he got this pneumonia. It was likely staphylococcus or streptococcus. The infection was no longer limited to his lungs; it had spread through his bloodstream. He had system-wide failure. The resulting vascular decompensation from his sepsis and dehydration complicated the picture. My knowledge of the pathophysiology was worth nothing. I could give a lecture on what was happening, but explanation didn't matter. My knowledge was useless. There was nothing I could do. I couldn't spin back time. The clock moved big forward, small back.

I looked back toward the patient. Still avoiding catching his mother's eye by accident. Sarah, arms stiff, delivered rhythmic and repetitive compressions. Our eyes locked with a silent exchange of information. She saw my frustration. My disbelief, really. My annoyance with myself and with God. She looked as though she had just seen a dog get hit by a car. The horror and confusion of your mind trying to rectify the things you see with what you believe.

I thought she might start to cry while she leaned over the boy. Pumping up and down, aggressively, unapologetically. She looked up to the clock, eyes glazed. She opened her mouth and exhaled slowly.

"Hey, Bruce, can you hang Rocephin? One hundred milligrams per kilogram." I turned to the patient again. "Sandy, give fifteen milliequivalents of bicarb and then another one point five milliliters of epinephrine. And I'm still waiting on his sugar?" I tried to slow the pace of my orders. I did this for me. Selfishly. This wasn't going to bring back PEA, a cardiac arrest. It wasn't going to bring back this boy. I just didn't want to face his mother. I didn't want to own up to my failure, my own fear of the void.

I turned my head back toward Bruce and his flood-worthy pants, "The labs are sent, right?" Bruce nodded back as he prepped the antibiotic. "Is that i-STAT coming anytime soon?" Still quiet, still annoyed.

"Coming." John, one of the techs, had been working on getting me the sugar with the i-STAT. There had been some sort of glitch delaying the result.

"Hold on." The small handheld i-STAT machine has a little horizontal bar across the bottom of the display window. It slowly blackens as the test approaches completion, just like waiting for a download on your computer.

"It says 110."

At least something is normal, I cynically said to myself. Placing my hand on the kid's carotid artery along the side of his neck, I said, "Hold CPR."

Again nothing.

"Continue CPR, please."

More slow-motion minutes passed. Selfish minutes. This kid was going to die. More accurately, he was dead.

I had recovered now, though. Somehow I had circled the void, but miraculously was able to bounce back to the present. I turned to the mom, ready to look her in the eye, the hospital chaplain now at her side. She was trembling, like she had just been immersed in an ice bath. She unknowingly picked at the edge of one thumb with the other. She didn't look at me, just stared at that highly polished linoleum floor.

"Looks like asystole," I said. Really, I was just telling the nurses I was getting ready to call it—the resuscitation was over. I was giving them a final chance to get their shit together as well. The monitor no longer showed the blips of electrical activity in the heart. There was nothing. Only a flat line.

Had I missed anything?

In vain, I was hoping the mom would know what *asystole* meant. As if this would somehow soften the blow that I was going to deliver.

Fuck me . . . again.

"Hand me the ultrasound." Taking the transducer, I pulled the monitor closer. The ultrasound would confirm that we were done.

From the day of birth till the day of death, your heart continually beats. It's one of the most amazing displays of endurance in all of physiology. The boy's race was over. His heart was motionless.

John, the ER tech, still held the i-STAT machine. I looked over at him and asked for the kid's potassium. I'm not even sure why I opened my mouth. But I asked anyway.

"Nine."

Normal potassium is around four. Nine is way off the scale of survivability. If Dr. Kevorkian wanted to help kill someone, potassium overdose would certainly be an option. For this little boy, the elevated potassium wasn't the cause of death. It was the result of his cells enduring too much. Without adequate oxygen and nutrients, the cells had succumbed to the overwhelming stress and broken open. This released a large amount of intracellular potassium into the extracellular space.

I didn't respond to the *nine*.

The silence was profound. The mother noted the pause and the quiet in the room. Like a panicked and caged animal, she suddenly sat upright in her chair, eyes darting back and forth. Like she was trying to find an escape from an impending zebra massacre. But there wasn't any.

I didn't want to know what she was feeling. I didn't want to share in her grief. I'm not a cold person. I just couldn't handle it. Even on the periphery, on the edge, it's too much.

I finally got her attention. Eye to eye, soul to soul. I gazed into a black hole leading to a different dimension. A dimension of emotion. Of fear, love, loss, and meaning. It was pure life.

In that moment, it felt like I saw too much. It made the hairs on the back of my neck stand on end. I was in a space that was vast, deep, and indescribable. I was there with her. I was her.

Opening my mouth made me sick. The sound of my voice made me sicker. But it didn't waver. The words came out solid and crisp.

She put her clenched fist over her mouth, trying to grab the air as it staccatoed its way out. Her body shook more vehemently. The pressure behind her eyes seemed too much. The black hole was closing. The dimension was folding in on itself. I fought back with my stare. Not because I wanted to, but because I had to.

If I close my eyes, I remember everything about that moment, every little detail. Her irises, the hair, her sweat, her breathing, and the smell of sepsis. I've heard you can remember faces better if you put them in context. I am well aware of the context, and her face is absolutely clear.

I looked up at the clock on the wall. Big forward, small back.

"Time of death, 8:12."

PART II

BAGPIPES

"Mull of Kintyre" Wings

The view was phenomenal. The water was deep blue, like a painter had used too much color. There was a subtle breeze; it felt fresh over my face, and I could see my wife's hair blowing back, like she was in a commercial for shampoo. In the distance, the Rocky Mountains stood off to the west, outlining the far edge of the lake.

The amphitheater was full; overflow attendees filled up the grassy knoll that extended upward beyond the benches. At least half of those attending were in uniform—flight suits, fire class As, paramedic whites, and military dress. People were mulling about, catching up, remembering old stories. But it all was slightly awkward.

I looked down at my watch. 11:00.

A silence came over the crowd.

The flight program members came in from the top of the amphitheater. Dark blue suits with orange stripes down the sleeves and legs. They walked in single file, quietly, solemnly. I stood at attention, not because I was told to, but because it felt necessary.

One by one, the flight team walked down the stairs until they reached the first and second rows in front of the stage. The entire program was in attendance and the processional was impressive.

The stage was also dramatic. A single casket sat in the middle. Flags on the edges. There were a few rows of chairs on either side of the coffin.

Following the flight crew came the military. They, too, were in their uniforms. They filed in with the efficiency of soldiers trained to form up and march. A few peeled off from the procession as it reached the bottom of the stairs. They made their way to the chairs that were on the stage.

Finally came the family of the dead; first the wife, then, with pomp and circumstance, at appropriate intervals, came the son, the grandchildren, and childhood friends. All the people who really mattered to him when he was living. One after another they took their positions on the stage.

A sharp but muted sound came from somewhere off to the right of the amphitheater stage, out of sight, some way off. I couldn't make out exactly what the voice said, but it barked an order. I could hear the faint rhythm of marching.

Earlier, when we arrived at the ceremony, there had been a traffic jam. Cops were at the intersections to help direct all the cars. So many people had descended on this small town, it was a bit overwhelmed.

Really, the memorial had started the day before. A motorcade had left St. Anthony's Hospital in Denver and made the sixty-mile trek up I-70 to Summit County. That is where the helicopter crash had happened. Ambulances, fire engines, emergency vehicles, and private cars had all made the drive together in a long single-file line. With the ambulance carrying the casket in the lead, they progressed slowly into the foothills. Lights flashing, they traveled with discipline and purpose. Lines of people stood on the roadside. Flags were draped on overpasses. I saw the weighty images on the news.

As we pulled up to the intersection at Lake Dillon, a policeman flagged us over. The main parking lot was full. We were instructed to go to overflow parking or find a spot in the nearby shopping center.

People were everywhere, but I was lucky enough to find a spot near a Starbucks. We ran across the street to get on the path that circumvented the lake. As we walked over the rise, Lake Dillon came into view. It was beautiful.

We drive by it all the time on our way to ski. It is a key waypoint when deciding which resort to hit. Continue on I-70 past the lake and you'll arrive at Copper Mountain and then Vail. If you take the exit and wrap around the southern end of the lake you'll be on your way to A-Basin, Keystone, or Breckenridge.

Today I realized that for all the times I've driven by the lake, I'd never stopped and gotten out of the car. I'd never taken the time to enjoy the beauty of this specific location.

My wife told me she used to camp here. I could see why.

We walked along the east bank. The crisp mountain air smelled wonderful. The rise forced me to breathe a little heavier. You never totally acclimatize to the altitude. We chatted as we walked. The crowd thickened as we made our way to the ceremony.

The path dropped a little, then rose again. As we came around the final curve we saw two fire trucks, both with big buckets on extended and telescoping ladders. A giant American flag hung between them. A Boy Scout troop had come out to line the pathway. They also held American flags. The wind blew perfectly, causing them to ripple and point toward the entrance of the amphitheater.

This would make a perfect wedding venue. I would have loved to have had my wedding here. It is majestic. Colorado is one of the most beautiful states in the country. I've spent a lot of time working in Europe and traveling across the US, and I've been exposed to some of the world's best views. Yet whenever I come home, I'm reminded of how lucky I am.

Today's scenic panorama wasn't for a wedding.

Helicopter Emergency Medical Services (HEMS) is a vital part of our medical system. It is like the special forces of the medical system. When distance, speed, and the critical nature of a patient require special attention, the helicopter and crew launch into action.

I started my medical career working as an EMT on an ambulance in California. The service was called RELS. Redwood Empire Life Support. The parent company also owned and operated a helicopter, REACH. Redwood Empire Air Care Helicopter. Quality acronyms.

The first time I saw the helicopter land I was mesmerized. The thing was so loud and powerful. It maneuvered into position over the landing site and then slowly touched down. I'm sure I was standing there smiling. Probably with my mouth open. Which is a little bit of a problem when you're taking care of a supersick patient that required a helicopter.

I thought the helicopter was rad. I thought the crew was even cooler. They were like gods. Everyone knows that they should dial 911 when they are in trouble. But when EMS shows up and they become overwhelmed, they call the helicopter. It is like the rescue for the rescue.

The first day I saw REACH land, we were taking care of a guy who was really messed up from an auger. It was that day that I knew I wanted to work on a medical helicopter. I wanted to be the rescue for the rescue.

I should probably clarify. I knew but I didn't. Like that is any clarification. My life has never followed a straight line, and my path to emergency medicine was no exception. Let's just say that at the time, I didn't know. But when I look back now, I did. More on that later.

Sorry, I tend to get distracted. Sitting in my seat watching the funeral, I heard another verbal order and then noticed the continued unified gait of the formation. The marching became louder and louder as the group moved down the path. I first saw the tops of the Glengarry caps and the tips of the pipes. Then the dark uniforms. Different plaids representing different families and histories. Some blue-and-green with subtle lines, others red with choppy squares. The heads bobbed in unison. I could hear the sequential drop of their feet, moving closer to the inevitable.

They passed under the same American flag hung between the fire trucks and stopped just short of the entrance, patrolling in place.

My wife leaned over and whispered, "Oh jeez, bagpipers."

She's a firefighter. You may not know this, but firefighters and bagpipers have a special connection. It's related to their mortality, running into dangerous situations, and having bagpipers show up to the ramifications of their heroism. Meaning, when a firefighter dies, bagpipers often give a voice to their heroism at the funeral.

The leader shouted another order. The color guard shifted as the handheld American flag dropped slightly and then moved forward. The pipers started to play. There is a raw emotion to the bagpipe, a yearning for attention. It's full of reflection and reverence. You can hear the pipes' desire to sound off, to make you believe.

F-15

"Top Gun Anthem" Harold Faltermeyer

I never planned on going to medical school. I wanted to be a fighter pilot. And I don't mean just like every other boy who saw *Top Gun*. I really, really wanted to be a fighter pilot.

Starting about seven years old, I began to home in on making it a reality. I had books on fighters that I memorized and could recite verbatim. Posters and models covered my room. By thirteen I was sure I wanted to go to the Air Force Academy. Again, this wasn't some whimsical determination. I had actually interviewed different military members—Navy sailors, Air Force airmen, and Marines, all friends of my parents—to find out the best landing spot for a would-be pilot. Strange behavior for sure. If I had any doubt that I could make it, I tried to temper it by working harder and more fervently toward my goal. Looking at my own kids, I realize I was a bit weird. I don't think I was a normal thirteen-year-old.

From the moment I entered high school, I was driven in my preparation, not only for selection to the Academy, but onward to an F-15 Eagle. The F-16 Falcon was a close second. My father always told me I could do whatever I wanted, and my mother backed it up with a calm *I'll-always-be-there* kind of peaceful, ever-available presence. And I believed them. If I put my mind to it and worked hard enough, I could achieve anything.

During my senior year of high school, I sat down in the front of seven or eight chairs, ready for my panel-style interview with Senator Cranston. To go to the Air Force Academy you not only need to be accepted to the school, you also need an appointment from a senator or congressman. I needed this to go well if I were going to make it.

They asked a series of questions about my life and how I got here. Typical interview items. I remember one portion of the interview particularly well. One of the panel members asked me, "What would you say if we told you that you had to fly an F-111?"

Now, the Aardvark (the F-111) is no Eagle, but still, I knew all about it. I rattled off some stats and made some comments about swept wings and General Dynamics, showing them that I knew my stuff. I ended by telling them that it was one of the most complicated airplanes to fly. And that was absolutely fine with me. I was up for the challenge.

As I stood up to leave my interview, the panel lead gave me some parting words. "When you get home, let you parents know that you did very, very well."

On Day One, I stepped off the bus in Colorado Springs, caught in an absolute whirlwind. It felt like mayhem.

Cadets and soldiers were screaming at the tops of their lungs, telling me to go here, stand over there, buzz my hair off, fill out this form, grab my gear, shut up, march, run, assume the push-up position.

The Air Force Academy was completely overwhelming. No matter how much you mentally prepare, I don't think you ever know until you're there, on the grounds, nervous, excited, tired, and confused. That is life at the Academy. In fact, that's the purpose of the Academy: to prepare you for the cluster of war. It is designed to train you to think under pressure, not freeze. It trains you to have clarity when others have panic. Steady. Solid. Quiet hands.

Daily life as a doolie, or first-year cadet, is a bombardment of agitation and stress. It builds you as a person and a soldier. Building character sucks, especially when you're actually building character.

I thought I had made it. As I closed my eyes for some fitful sleep that first night, I heard my roommate take a deep breath. I felt the same. Exhausted, I needed rest, but I was so fired up to finally have made it. I thought I was going to be a fighter pilot.

I don't know if this has happened to you, but it happens to me all the time. I get caught up in the romantic view of things. I fail to spend any considerable time on the realistic view. In my romantic view, the Academy was flashy and sexy. I was going to breeze through. I'd be like the picture you see in the brochure—self-assured, tough, proud. The realistic view was more mundane and sullen. I would be a bookworm, wound up, stressed, squaring corners, and eating meals with my fork at 90 degrees.

I also get caught up in the entry, but don't focus enough on the exit. What I mean is, I get so focused on just getting to my goal. And my naïve self doesn't know the real goal. It's a picturesque journey that doesn't necessarily have all the nitty-gritty and troublesome parts. I thought the Academy was the goal and being a fighter pilot was an afterthought, gravy on top of the mashers. One followed the other, like the "given" in geometry. But then, as if it's a surprising turn of events, I realize that the goal in my head may not have been the endpoint.

The first night lying at the Academy, I was thinking about being a fighter pilot. I wasn't thinking about the four years of college, then flight school, then aircraft selection, and everything else in between. The process in front of me, in and of itself, was a significant chunk of my life. I had focused on getting to a moment, a cadet trying to fall asleep in my dorm room. That was my tangible. I figured the rest would fall into place.

The first time I rode my bike was glorious. I had tried, just like every other kid, to keep it upright, over and over. This was before there were Striders. Striders are an amazing invention, an innovation really, that crosses a scooter with a bike. The genius is in one simple modification. They just took the pedals and cranks off. This lets the kid put their feet on the ground so they feel solid and secure. They get a feel for moving forward on a bike without ever abandoning the safety of the ground. But I digress.

The first time I started to cruise on my bike, a real bike with cranks and pedals, I was ecstatic. Riding on my own was remarkable. It is one of the best moments of my life. The freedom, exhilaration, and excitement all flowed together, like the Ghostbusters crossing the streams at a single point in time and space. I was a kid, but I felt like a god. I was in control. I could go wherever I wanted, however fast I wanted. It opened an entirely new world. One that was larger and brighter than ever before.

That utter sense of invincibility ultimately ends, though. Every novice bike rider knows that. It's pretty much part of the deal. If you ride a bike, eventually gravity is going to win, even with angular momentum on your side. I don't think there was a chunk of the summer that I wasn't covered in some sort of road rash—or poison oak (but that's a different story).

One particularly stellar accident sticks out in my mind. It happened midsummer, deep enough in that I had a routine but not far enough through that I had become bored with the repetitive nature of the carefree days. My friends and I had just finished a neighborhood baseball game. As with most of these games, it ended with some amount of emotional distress and an argument over a missed or bad call. I don't remember who, but one of us had been blatantly wronged and we were breaking up until at least the next morning.

My friend's house was about a quarter mile away, up the hill on a dirt road to the right. We lived on Bones Road in Sebastopol. It was in the boondocks. And yes, it was truly called Bones Road. About a mile away, on the same street, was a hippie school called Nonesuch. Again, no lie. They taught tie-dye, weaving, and farming.

I huffed away from the unfair baseball game and jumped on my BMX. I rocketed down the hill like usual, like a fighter pilot. First a left, then a right with a steeper grade past the walnut tree. Another hundred feet, and I ripped a right to head through the gate into our driveway.

Unperceived by me, there was a thin wire strung up horizontally between the two posts. It was about two feet off the ground. A white line was painted on the pavement below it. This line had been painted and the wire subsequently placed for our dogs. My dad had read that he could train the dogs to stay in the yard by stringing an electric fence through the gaps. The dogs couldn't detect the wire, he said, so he painted a white stripe on the ground. The dogs would equate the white line with the shock. Soon, you could forgo the wire and only have the white stripe. Voila, our dogs would never leave the premises.

I suspect you see where this is going. I knew about the white line and the dogs and all that. The only problem is that my dad hadn't deployed the wire for about a year. This meant that I, as a kid, completely disregarded the threat of the wire and the underlying white line. (The dogs crossed the line too. So I wasn't alone, just saying). I came tearing through the gate, took that hard right, and the front tire met the wire head-on. You can imagine my surprise. The bike suddenly stopped cold, like hitting an invisible wall (or in this case an invisible wire). My body continued forward, and I flew like Superman. But not the kind of Superman I dreamed about. There was no sustained lift. Just a pull, nine meters per second squared downward.

I hit hard, rolled, and then slid. There is a moment when you crash and realize you've crashed, but the pain hasn't set in yet. It's like a moment of Zen.

I like when seven-year-olds swear (although I wouldn't admit it to my kids). After the impact and slide, I immediately jumped up. In part to prove that I wasn't dead and in part because I was so freakin' pissed. My mom and dad had both been out in the front yard working. They had seen the whole thing. I remember specifically not looking at my dad but shouting, "Who in the hell strung up that wire!" My mom immediately screamed something more profound, but I won't repeat it here. I'm sure my dad remembers.

Then the pain set in. Moment of Zen over. I bent in half, cradling my road-rashed arm and bruised elbow. That quickly yielded to the pain in my right knee. And my left. I looked like I was wearing a plaid red jumpsuit, which I wasn't, just to clarify.

Man, that hurt.

I remember sitting on the airplane flying home from the Academy. I looked out the window over the desert and felt sad. I was a washout. Someone who didn't complete the four years. I wasn't in the Air Force anymore. I wasn't going to be a fighter pilot. I had been completely goal-oriented without a backup plan. I was in unfamiliar territory. And what's more, I deserved it. I really thought that. Because I cheated myself to get there.

There are moments in everyone's life where you wish you had a redo. I needed a mulligan, but it wasn't at the Academy like you might be thinking. It was before.

During preparation for acceptance to the Academy, you're put through the gauntlet, not just academically, but physically. I drove to Sacramento from my hometown of Sebastopol for my medical evaluation. I was a healthy high school varsity athlete. I felt great and was fully expecting to pass with flying colors. Just the next stepping-stone on my way to the F-15.

Everything had been going perfectly until I got to the eye exam. After some preliminary checks, I was moved into a room with a vision chart. I sat down in the mechanical chair and looked at the chart. Nothing out of the ordinary, I thought. That was until the doc covered up my right eye and asked me which line I could read. I started out EDFCZP, no problem. He asked if I could read the line below. That was going to be an issue. It was blurry as hell. FEL, or was it EFL? I couldn't tell. I struggled to start, sitting on the first letter for a bit.

Just then, someone stuck their head in the room and asked the doc to step out for a second. He gave a quick, well-meaning grunt and got up from his chair. I opened both eyes, leaned forward and checked out the chart. Using both eyes, squinting, and leaning forward, I could make out the line I was on and the one below, barely. FELOPZD, DEFPOTEC. I wasn't going to pass the eye exam. At the time, pilots needed 20/20 vision. There were no waivers, and corrected vision didn't count. No glasses, contacts, or procedures. LASIK wasn't even available.

In a complete moment of panic, I realized my goal of becoming a pilot was going to end in this eye exam chair.

This is where I want the mulligan.

It is where I realized that life isn't always fair. It is where I learned that I wasn't who I wanted to be. I wasn't as good as they all thought.

Sitting forward in my chair, I memorized the chart. I mean I literally, in the span of ten seconds, memorized every line of the eye chart.

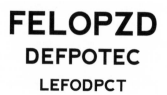

FELOPZD
DEFPOTEC
LEFODPCT

I cheated.

The doctor came back in. I rattled off the requested line and the next smaller line. I passed without issue. Cleared for the Academy.

I thought it was a fluke. Maybe it was the shirt and tie cutting off circulation to my brain. I reasoned that I was just tired, that my eyes were having a bad day. I hadn't noticed my eyes were going bad in normal life, so this just had to be a little speed bump that almost threw my car off the road. Fortunately, I overcame and adapted, exactly what they wanted in a cadet. That's how I worked it out. That's how I felt good about myself. I created my reality. But it was fake.

The funny thing is, at the Air Force Academy, they recheck your eyes. The entrance exam is not the only eye exam on the agenda.

PING-PONG

"Sooner or Later" Mat Kearney

About halfway through my last year of college at UC Davis, I came to a fairly sudden conclusion. It wasn't my idea. I think it was my roommate Dave's idea, but I don't even remember for sure. He pointed out that I liked being an EMT. My cycling coach was an MD, and I always commented on the interesting physiology of training. Dave knew I didn't want to be an economist or work as a business guy. "Why don't you be a doctor? You're good in school. You'd probably like it." Dave wanted to be a doctor, too, so maybe his advice was biased.

I should back up just a little. And by a little, I mean about four years. I left the Academy and enrolled at UC Davis.

I left the Academy of my own free will. And by left, I mean I quit. I was a quitter because I couldn't deal with the fact that I wasn't going to fly the F-15, or any aircraft for that matter. There are plenty of career opportunities for an

Air Force Academy graduate besides flying, but not for me. If I couldn't have it my way, then I wasn't staying.

That decision has stuck with me my entire life. That lame-ass mindset cost me years of sleepless nights. Because of my weakness and stubbornness, my inability to comprehend my lack of control, I internally became—and subsequently deemed myself—a quitter. No matter what I would do, or the successes I would have, I could never overcome my own disdain for this perceived failing when I left the Academy. But more on that later.

Back to UC Davis. Why Davis? Mainly because that is where both my best friend and my girlfriend went to school. Also, the dean let me transfer in from the Academy directly. I didn't have to go through the typical application process. I'd like to say there was more to it, but that wouldn't be true. Having been driven so long, I was out of my element when I flew home on that airplane. I was at a loss. To be honest, I didn't think much of myself. No one else would have noticed. My girlfriend and buddy probably didn't know, but that is what I thought.

I switched my major from aeronautical engineering to economics. I couldn't handle talking about and studying airplanes. I'd switch to supply and demand. Widgets were simpler and less emotional, for me, at least.

My parents must have been panicking a little. They had been lucky enough to have had a motivated kid who wanted to go to the Air Force Academy. That had kept me focused and on the straight and narrow. When I returned home, they had to worry that I would go off the deep end. And little did they know I was standing on the end of the diving board. Like so much in life, I was able to hide things on the outside. I would save up my demons for the night.

When I was alone and couldn't outwit my knowledge of the truth.

I have five rules for my kids. I repeat them over and over, ad nauseam, as they would attest.

1. No pregnancy.
2. No drugs.
3. Don't drink and certainly don't drink and drive.
4. Play a sport.
5. Try hard in school.

These rules can be summed up even further by my wife: No births, no deaths.

So even though I had dropped out of the Academy, I was abiding by my rules. OK, mostly. I was still in college, so I might have had a beer or two.

But those rules were easy to follow. What I was struggling with was my emotional self. I struggled with what the people on the outside saw, and what I thought about myself on the inside. The two notions seemed to contradict each other. I struggled with a panic, a yet-to-be-accepted notion of reality. That life went on, regardless of my intentions. That no matter how hard I tried, or how much I wanted something, I was really not in control. My efforts to manipulate my surroundings resulted in only an illusion of control.

For so many years I had known exactly what I wanted to do. I had thought I knew exactly what I needed to do to get there. But now, I was a new me. A different me. I floated around the economics building showing diligence and hard work, but I had no fire. I had all the excitement of

Helen Keller in an art gallery. That may sound a little dark, but I thought it. So there it is. I can't help it sometimes.

On a whim, I signed up for an EMT course. It was offered at Davis through the outdoor ed program. I thought it might be a cool summer job, driving around on an ambulance. At least better than flipping burgers, to my mind.

Every week on Wednesday night I would come to class and studiously listen to my instructor. I thought he was a genius. I was drinking the Kool-Aid. Sure, I would work hard on my economics studies because I wasn't stupid. If I didn't get good grades in college, my folks wouldn't be so liberal with the tuition. But the EMT class—that I studied because I thought it was cool.

I remember my first patient interactions. My pulse would go so high. I'd act as if it truly were *my* emergency, in addition to *their* emergency. I think the stress drew me in because it offered a rush, and I liked it. Moments of panic, when someone is freaking out, that's when it is time to step in and save the day. It gave me a sense of purpose, more than any supply/demand curve or tariff calculation. And I think economics is great. Really, I do. I use what I learned from my economics degree daily. That probably speaks to the sad state of healthcare. But for my personality, I just couldn't see doing economics as a full-time gig.

I finished EMT school and immediately applied for a summer job on an ambulance. For my first interview, I ended up at the wrong company's headquarters. I was confused why they had no idea who I was and why they looked at me blankly when I said I had an interview. My bad.

It was *such* a surprise when I didn't get the job. But I wasn't going to let that stop me. The next interview went a bit better. I made sure I had the right company, for starters.

I spent the summer logging a ton of hours, because that's what EMTs and paramedics do. They work like crazy, in part because the pay sucks. Also, because it becomes an identity. And yeah, running a good call is like crack.

It is also a great job for an individual who bores easily and probably has a diagnosis of ADHD or some variant. I've never taken medicine or anything, but I'm sure everyone around me thinks I'm a bit of a squirrel.

Now that I've admitted I have something like ADHD, you have to bear with me for one more jump.

When I came to UC Davis, I started to race bicycles. UC Davis is a huge bike school. Everyone rides their bike everywhere. And they had a very good competitive cycling team.

Racing gave me the same freedom I had when I first started to ride my bike. It also gave me a chance to deal with my inner demons. Racing a bike hard, to the limit, you can really test yourself. You know when you've had enough, and you know when you've pushed through the moment you thought you had had enough. It was almost like I wanted to torture myself with the suffering on the bike. In some sick way, I liked it. I wanted the pain. I wanted the suffering.

I also wanted to prove to myself that I wasn't a quitter. Because no matter what I did, it was never enough.

I remember during my first big weekend group ride with the team, we started to climb a long and steep ascent. Soon, one by one, team members started to drop off. Toward the summit, the team captain looked around. There were only a few of us left. He rode next to me and said, "Who are you?"

"I'm Shannon!" Like that meant something to him.

"I mean, what category are you racing?" he asked.

"Ds."

In collegiate racing there are categories A–D, A being the fastest, D being the slowest. Since I had never raced before I assumed I was a D.

"Not for long," was all he said as he turned up the pace for the final kilometer of the climb. He dropped me . . . but I didn't quit. He seemed surprised to see me crest the summit not too far off his pace.

This leads me to where I started the chapter: my final year of college and the best roommates ever.

Dave had made a straightforward suggestion. Nothing profound. He said it simply. "Why don't you be a doctor? You're good in school. You'd probably like it."

I started to mull it over. I would like it. Clearly, this was what I was meant to do. This would settle my unrest. This had to be the reason that the Academy didn't work out. God must have had a plan. If I became a doctor, then I wouldn't be a failure or a quitter. Being a doctor would show that the fighter pilot thing was just a misguided plan.

I had taken the EMT class on a whim, and that decision introduced me to medicine. Now Dave's suggestion became my conclusion. I was going to be a doctor.

I loved working on the ambulance. It was a perfect setup to be a hero. People called and you answered. You never knew what was around the next corner and had to be prepared for anything. It was stressful but rewarding. Maybe it would allow me to prove something to myself.

Being a doctor put you in the heat of battle. Not to mention, you got to work with helicopters now and again when things really got jacked up.

Dave was totally right. But I wasn't entirely sure what being a doctor entailed. There are no doctors in my family. I didn't have any close mentors or friends who were doctors, but from the outside it seemed pretty good. Respectable and exciting work. I had stumbled out of aeronautical engineering, into economics, and now was taking a left turn to become a doctor. It made perfect sense, to me.

So although I didn't know much about being a doctor, I felt like this was the right move. I also was gravitating toward emergency medicine, even before I started to apply. It would be just like the ambulance but better.

The first meeting with a premed advisor stressed me out. She had a superiority complex and seemed to enjoy making me doubt any chance of my success. "You're a bit behind the eight ball," were the first words out of her mouth after looking over my file.

Of course I am, I thought. As I just mentioned, I wanted to be a pilot, failed, studied economics, and now I'm planning on medicine. Sounds like the perfect doctor candidate. *Not.*

She went on to explain my situation and timeline. As an economics major, aside from math, I didn't have any of the prerequisites. I'd have to do an extra year and a half of "postbac" to finish chemistry, organic chemistry, physics, and biology. I'd then have to wait for the next cycle of the MCAT (Medical College Admission Test). Only after getting my results could I apply in the fall to matriculate the following year. Best-case scenario? I'd be entering medical school two and half years after this initial meeting.

I sat quietly in my chair, processing the newly acquired information. My advisor looked at me with a bit of skepticism and shrugged. She seemed to be saying, *Go ahead and try to get in if you want to. It's your life. Don't blame me if no one takes you.* She certainly didn't see me as one of her stronger candidates, and she had no problem letting me know it.

I rode home on my dilapidated beach cruiser bike that was painted like a cow, pink udder and all (UC Davis's unofficial mascot is a cow), thinking about the meeting. By the time I walked in the front door I was pissed. *I'm going to prove her wrong,* I thought to myself.

I harnessed my angst from quitting the Academy. No way was I going to give up. No way was I going to quit this process, even if my adviser seemed to think that I should stop before I started. I also knew that I wanted to do this right. I wanted to earn it, on my own. I never wanted to feel the emotions of leaving the Academy again. I would never compromise who I am for where I wanted to be. It just isn't worth it. That's what I decided. *And who is she to tell me I can't make it?*

I was going to have to work my ass off. I was clearly behind, but a goal that isn't potentially out of reach isn't a goal at all. I'd have to put some oomph into this one. I was pissed not only because she doubted me, but also because I felt like she was partially right. Maybe I wouldn't be able to make it. Maybe I would quit even if I didn't want to. Maybe she really was an advisor and I just didn't like her advice.

I heard a familiar racket out back, and I walked outside to tell my roommates what had happened. They were in the middle of an intense ping-pong match to determine who would wash all the dishes.

"Well, that sucked. She said I'd be lucky to get in," I announced as I plopped down in the lawn chair.

My roommate Richie said, "Lame!"

Still keeping his attention on the game, another room-mate, Jon, smiled. "OK, you play me next game. If you win we'll both get in med school. If I win, you do the dishes and I still get in." With that, he attempted to slam a crosscourt shot, which just missed the edge of the table. And yes, I'm well aware that more than one of my roommates wanted to be a doctor.

Oh, he didn't want any part of my ambidextrous ping-pong playing right now. Had he not seen I was fired up? I sat fuming while Richie and Jon finished their game. When my turn came up, I proceeded to light Jon up in one of our standard best-of-five matches. When we finished, he jok-ingly grimaced and said, "She did fire you up." With that, he flipped his paddle on the table and strutted off toward the kitchen like he was in a rap video. "Fine. I guess now we're *both* going to medical school," he said, laughing, as the screen door slammed behind him.

"And you're doing the dishes." My voice trailed off as he failed to look back.

Jon's now a surgeon in California. That ping-pong table was something special. I should also mention that my other roommate, Dave, who gave me the great idea, never became a doctor. He joined the Navy to become a pilot. Now, that's weird. That table . . . something special.

Two years later, after busting my butt, I walked into the same counselor's office and showed her what I had done. I had killed my classes and aced the MCAT. Remarkably (sarcasm), she had suddenly become the best advisor ever.

"I haven't seen *that* MCAT score before." She stared at the paper. "Let's see what we can do."

I wondered where the "we" had come from, as if there had been a "we" when I was pulling an all-nighter studying for my O-Chem final or trying to finish my gazillion-page physiology lab research paper. Now that my counselor thought I had a shot at getting into the big leagues, she was all over me like flies on a rib roast, like she worked on commission or something.

The first meeting she had made me edgy and uncomfortable by pointing out my presumed weakness; now she made me uncomfortable with her overconfidence and readiness to jump on my bandwagon, albeit a slightly delayed one. The roles had reversed. At first, she was skeptical of me, and now I was skeptical of her. Excellent MCAT scores and four-point-oh grades do not guarantee anything in med school admissions.

I'm a bit superstitious in that I had learned not to count my chickens before they hatched. I might have realized that from *not* being a fighter pilot. But that's what she was doing over there—counting my chickens—and it made me nervous. I knew the competition, and it was frightfully smart and tough. I needed to look no further than any of my current lab partners. They were straight A students with extensive research and medically related backgrounds. Two of the three played scholarship athletics, and all three had already published something. The admissions process would be challenging. I still had my work cut out for me.

HELL YEAH!

"My Songs Know What You Did in the Dark" Fall Out Boy

Columbia University in New York City is awe inspiring. I arrived for my interview mesmerized by its history and reputation. This place was old-school, really old-school, and I don't mean that in some East Coast/West Coast rapper lingo. Founded in 1754 by royal charter of King George II, it exuded a pride and tradition I felt the moment I arrived. Columbia is one of the top medical schools in the country, and, like my counselor pointed out in our first meeting, I couldn't help but wonder if I was out of my league.

It was a far cry from where I grew up. I can tell you that Columbia is distant, both physically and philosophically, from Nonesuch, the school of my homeland. As I walked through the stoned carved arches, I gave myself a quick and silent pep talk.

I managed to repress my self-doubt as I began the first of three interviews. *Tell me a little about yourself.* And so the process started.

I settled into my chair and hunkered down for any verbal melee that might ensue, but fortunately it never did. Aside from the fact that my bladder seemed to suddenly have a 90 percent decrease in its usual capacity, the interviews were quite mellow and nonstressful. The interviewers, various specialists from Columbia's medical faculty, although formal, seemed to be friendly and truly interested in my responses to their questions. They didn't pose any of the odder or more annoying questions I had encountered elsewhere, like "If there was static on your TV, what would it be?" *Thanks, Oregon. What would it be? I don't even know what the heck you're talking about.*

The questions from Columbia were more direct and uncomplicated. We talked about bike racing, music, and where I grew up. The interviews felt more like normal conversations, and the time passed quickly. Before I knew it, I was shaking hands with my last interviewer and heading back to the waiting area. *That was pretty painless,* I thought.

After a short wait, four Columbia students came to take us on a tour. They had volunteered to show us around during their lunch break and give us the inside scoop on student life. It felt totally laid back. One of the students, Mike, asked me how my interviews went.

"Did you have Dr. Landry?" he asked.

"Yeah," I said, nodding.

"He's the best teacher. Hilarious. That guy should have been a comedian."

I thought to myself, *Teachers that are comedians—that's what I'm talkin' about.* I walked around and liked everything about the school—top-notch facilities, cool students, funny teachers, and New York City. It couldn't get much better than this. Columbia seemed like the place for me. As I drove away, sitting on the bench seat of the yellow cab, I glanced back at the huge medical complex. I got excited. Man, I wanted to go to Columbia. Hopefully, I had convinced them that I should be in their next first-year class.

After returning home, I reviewed all the applicant material from the various schools where I had interviewed. I kept coming back to the Columbia brochure; it made me nervous, itchy nervous. I didn't want to miss out on this opportunity so I decided to write a letter to Dr. Frantz, the dean of admissions. I hadn't met Dr. Frantz during my interview, and I knew that was a bit of a problem. But I had a plan. I'd tell him how awesome his school is and how much I wanted to attend. I'd tell him that I was the perfect candidate. This would likely cause him to personally look over my application and see that I was exactly what Columbia was looking for.

That's how it played out in my mind.

In the letter, I offered to fly out for a second round of interviews to help him make his decision.

Each day I checked the mail for a response; it was excruciating. I'm talking about snail mail, not email. Finally, two weeks later I saw the Columbia University seal as I peered into the mailbox. I tore the envelope open right then and there, standing at the end of Bones Road, and anxiously read. I was reasonably sure that it was a positive letter, but Dr. Frantz's capacious vocabulary made me feel like I was reading a passage from the verbal section of the SAT. I honestly had to pull out the dictionary when I got home just to assure myself that I had understood his meaning. Although he had some "arrière-pensée" because he could promise me nothing, my "alacrity" to come only increased my chances. Albeit slim chances, considering I couldn't even communicate with the dean of admissions without consulting Webster's.

He had placed the ball back in my court, at least as far as I could tell from my scholarly interpretation. The lack of funds in my checking account caused me a bit of stress, but I surely needed to make the trip. I had suggested the whole idea so it would look idiotic not to follow through. Besides, my sister and brother-in-law lived in nearby Greenwich, Connecticut. If you know of Greenwich you're probably asking yourself why they didn't just pay for me to visit. They lived in Greenwich but were hired help. Teachers by day, nannies by night. There was more of a chance that I could get Mom and Dad to pitch in not only for the interview but also for a "sister-brother bonding trip."

I arrived at the interview nervous but focused. I liked interviews, believe it or not, and I knew I was going to have to roll this one up and smoke it. I also showed up at the right address, so that was a plus. After checking in with the secretary, I sat in the small reception area. I quickly reexamined my appearance: tie straight, shirt tucked, fly up, straight gig line, and no stray hair from my sister's cat. Thank you, Air Force.

After a brief wait, the secretary escorted me into Dr. Frantz's office. I passed through a large room that housed all the "ladies" who handled the admission process. I felt their eyes fall upon me. The venerable Dr. Frantz met me just outside his door. I had seen him from a distance during my first visit but, as I said, hadn't met him. I took note of his frail, crooked appearance. His scapula winged outward, and he stood kind of cockeyed, with one shoulder higher than the other. He wore his ever-present white coat, gray slacks, and a P&S tie—always a P&S tie. With his hic-coughed gait, he ambled back into his office, with me following close at his heels.

The next thirty minutes passed in a flash. We had a great conversation that eventually came to the topic of literature. He was a lover of fiction and had an expansive knowledge. I had just finished reading *Flowers for Algernon* by Daniel Keyes. I had read it, in large part—OK, in total part—for the interview process. Somewhere in some "interviewing like a champ" book, I had read that they may ask me what book I was reading. I didn't want to respond with *MAD Magazine*, so I read *Flowers*. You have to try to put the odds in your favor.

He asked, "What did you think of it?"

I thought for a moment. I really did like it. It's one of my favorite books, just after *Foucault's Pendulum* and *Ender's Game*. "Charlie is happy when the book starts out. He's naïve to the cruel nature of the world. When he becomes 'smart,' he becomes self-aware." I thought for a moment longer. "Knowledge and intelligence, and success for that matter, don't equal happiness." I said it like I believed it. Which, at the time, I'm not sure I did.

Dr. Franz paused and then responded, "True . . . and intellectual aptitude does not equate to emotional intelligence. Happiness comes from within, rather than some external expectation." Dr. Frantz asked, "Do you like Walker Percy?"

I felt a wave of panic because I couldn't remember what he had written—my high school English teacher would have been disappointed . . . again.

Fortunately, he continued before I revealed my igno-
rance. "He attended Columbia, you know. We have a
Walker Percy society." I took note that at a place like
Columbia, nobody used the word *club* when they could use
the word *society*.

As he looked over my résumé, he remarked, "So, you
play soccer."

"Yes, sir."

I haven't mentioned that I played soccer, but I did. In
high school and at the Air Force Academy. After I left the
Academy, I never played for UC Davis's team. Never even
tried out. I think that was part of my whole identity issue
when I left school in Colorado Springs. But I will tell you
this: along with my buddies Dave and Mike, our rec team,
in open league, beat the UC Davis soccer team in intramu-
ral competition. The picture is on the wall of the activity
center to prove it! It wasn't the official UC Davis Soccer
Team with the uniforms and all, but it was all the players
from the team, and I'll count it.

"Soccer players are usually pretty fast."

I smirked slightly.

"Have you ever played rugby?"

"No, but it looks like fun." In reality, it looked dangerous.

I remembered not to answer with a negative. All good
interviewing guides tell you not to be negative. It's like
Disneyland. When the guest asks, "What time does the
park close?" the cast member responds in the positive: "The
Magic Kingdom stays open until nine." I had heard that Dr.
Frantz loved rugby and was fanatical about the Columbia
Medical School team. I wanted him to know that if playing
rugby would get me in, then I certainly couldn't wait to use

my speed, break my nose, or dislocate my shoulder for the good of Columbia rugby.

"We have a pretty good team here at Columbia. You should try and go to a game."

"I'd like that," I replied.

What transpired next totally caught me off guard. The room fell silent. Dr. Franz focused his gaze on me, as if trying to read my mind.

The clock moved. Big forward, small back.

After a brief moment, he seemed to have found what he was looking for. He leaned back in his leather chair and placed both hands on the edge of his desk.

"Well . . . ," he said, pausing for adequate effect. "I don't see any reason why you shouldn't come here. Do you?"

Shocked, I didn't know how to respond.

"Um, yes. I mean no. No reason I can see not to come here either." Double negatives always messed with me, especially at the Air Force Academy. I remember the commander would yell in my face, "You don't like me?" My options were *yes*, *no*, and *I don't understand*. None of these were good options. If I yelled, "Yes," he would say, "Yes, you don't like me?" If I said, "No," he would say, "No!!! You don't like me." And if I said, "I don't understand," he would just call me a fool.

Dr. Frantz stood and walked around the desk to shake my hand. "Of course you'll have to let all the other schools know you're coming to Columbia. We'll have you sign your acceptance paperwork out front."

Smiling in disbelief, I stood and shook his hand. His weren't construction-worker hands. They were the hands of an aged doctor. He led me out to his secretary, and she gave me a cuffed and smirk-like smile as I sat down in front of her desk. With no delay, she slid across an acceptance letter and pen.

Holy shit, he's serious.

She had the letter all ready. Do not pass go, do not collect two hundred dollars. It was my call, and I had to decide right now. No sleeping on it or discussing it with family. After only a brief pause, I let my signature flow, doctoresque, from the Columbia-logoed pen.

WHITE COAT

"All Along the Watchtower" Bob Dylan

The White Coat Ceremony occurs during orientation week, and it is a big deal at P&S, Columbia's College of Physicians and Surgeons. Begun by the Arnold P. Gold Foundation, it originated at our medical school in 1993. The foundation promoted humanism in medicine, and the White Coat Ceremony introduced students to the privilege and expectations of being a caring and compassionate physician. It represented the formal "cloaking" and "conversion" of laypeople into medical professionals, and initiated the new medical student into the medical fraternity.

Columbia takes the donning of the white coat very seriously. After that moment, the student's life changes forever. That's what they preached, anyway. Some diehards have likened it to taking a godly vow prior to joining the priesthood. I wouldn't go that far, but some doctors, including my dean, might. The ceremony displays the student's commitment to medicine. If it were possible,

Columbia probably would have preferred us branding our arms with a hot cauldron like in the beginning of the show *Kung Fu*—one side with a caduceus and the other with the Columbia crest. Since permanent disfigurement would likely cause a significant percentage of students to waver in their undying commitment, the white coat had to do.

Midway through the ceremony, we were all asked to stand. We were about to commence our indoctrination. Family, friends, and faculty were all present to witness this monumental event. I usually find "emotional" celebrations like the White Coat Ceremony a bit cheesy, but I have to admit, this one got me. As I stood there waiting to put on my lab coat, I basked in the glory of it all. I had finally made it to medical school. No more worrying about prerequisite grades, extracurricular activities, or MCAT scores. I was here. I looked side to side at all the faces of my classmates as we rose to take the Hippocratic Oath. They looked exactly how I felt. I joined in, and we all said, in unison:

> *I swear by Apollo the physician, by Esculapius, Hygeia, and Panacea, and I take to witness all the gods, all the goddesses, to keep according to ability and my judgment, the following Oath.*
>
> *To consider dear to me as my parents him who taught me this art; to live in common with him and if necessary to share my goods with him; to look upon his children as my own brothers; to teach them this art if they so desire without fee or written promise; to impart to my sons and the sons of the master who taught me and the*

disciples who have enrolled themselves and have agreed to the rules of the profession, but to these alone the precepts and the instruction.

I will prescribe regimens for the good of my patients according to my ability and my judgment and never do harm to anyone.

To please no one will I prescribe a deadly drug nor give advice which may cause his death.

Nor will I give a woman a pessary to procure abortion.

But I will preserve the purity of my life and my art.

I will not cut for stone, even for patients in whom the disease is manifest; I will leave this operation to be performed by practitioners, specialists in the art.

In every house where I come I will enter only for the good of my patients, keeping myself far from all intentional ill-doing and all seduction and especially from the pleasures of love with women and men, be they free or slaves.

All that may come to my knowledge in the exercise of my profession or in daily commerce with men, which ought not to be spread abroad, I will keep secret and will never reveal.

If I keep this oath faithfully, may I enjoy my life and practice my art, respected by all

*men and in all times; but if I swerve from it
or violate it, may the reverse be my lot.*

As the audience applauded, I slipped on my crisp white coat. It felt solid, compressed, and weighted. I wanted to become exactly what the Arnold P. Gold Foundation wished for me: a compassionate and scholarly healer. I remember my mom had tears in her eyes, and my dad smiled like he had just won a new car. *Man, this is going to be awesome.*

During the ceremony, Dr. Morgan, an internist and one of our curriculum advisors, took the podium. Her speech started like any standard welcoming address. With her head barely cresting the top of the lectern, she praised the school and honored all of us for making it through the arduous selection process. Parents and family members were duly thanked for their support and ongoing involvement. She continued talking for the next few minutes, and I tried to entertain myself by looking through the student handbook. I have a limited attention span.

I opened to the Arnold P. Gold Foundation section.

The Arnold P. Gold Foundation works with healthcare professionals in training and in practice to instill a culture of respect, dignity, and compassion for patients and professionals.

Humanistic medical care is not simply compassion. It is the best of medicine. When skilled physicians build caring, trusting, and collaborative relationships with patients, studies reveal more appropriate

*medical decisions, better patient adher-
ence with treatment plans, and less costly
healthcare outcomes.*

As I flipped forward to the student activity section, she regained my scrutiny with a notable change in her tone. I looked up. Her initial jovial and lighthearted voice had taken on a profound and diabolical quality. In a moment, she had the air of a priest giving a eulogy at a funeral. I was drawn in—pulled into some sinister moment—like in a thriller. As though my vision had telescoped in an instant, I found myself in an eye-to-eye confrontation with the speaker. Nothing and no one else existed.

Looking straight into my eyes, she said, "You want this? Are you ready for this?"

There was a prolonged caricature pause. Theatrical for effect, like Dr. Frantz. She continued to pierce me with her concentrated demon gaze, and I couldn't look away. Then it seemed as if a wave of sadness came over her. She seemed to show empathy, compassion, love, and finally hope. Turning from demon to angel, softly she said, "Your innocence will be lost . . . forever."

Big forward, small back.

As fast as it all started, it ended. It was a weird experience, very weird. Maybe I imagined it. But I don't think so. The auditorium returned to normal. Time started moving again.

PART III

AUTOROTATION

"Wheels" Foo Fighters

've never been a pallbearer. It's not like being a best man, something you'd want to do. I scanned the group of bag-pipers. An ambulance pulled up behind them. Silently, the lights spun. It sat at the entrance to the right of the stage.

The wail of the bagpipes stopped, and I noted that six men of varying statures, wearing dark suits, walked up to the back of the ambulance as the attendant opened the door. Purposefully they slid out the casket and grabbed the handles. It looked heavy.

The pallbearers moved slowly and deliberately. The coffin was closed, for obvious reasons. They placed it on a trolley in front of the stage, and a religious cloth, white and gold, was laid over the top.

Pat Mahany's wife and family were on the stage. It's voyeurism to watch the family at a funeral. They ema-nate pure emotion. It's the type of emotion that is usually private, should be private, but on the stage, with the beautiful Lake Dillon backdrop, it was displayed for everyone.

Pat's wife stood up and walked over to the priest. They exchanged a few words. She was handed a grey helmet. She clutched it like she didn't want to let it go. Then, after a few moments, she set it in front of the casket.

It wasn't really his helmet. At least not the one from the crash. It looked too good.

Every time the helicopter takes off, there can be consequences. There is an inherent danger to flying, especially in helicopters. It's not a forgiving endeavor.

Flying in Colorado doesn't make things any easier. The altitude of the Rocky Mountains and the rapidly changing weather all add to the challenge.

In HEMS, the risk is mitigated by exhaustive training, endless regulations, and meticulous attention to detail. We have highly trained, highly competent pilots with thousands of hours behind the stick. The medical crew members receive intensive training on crew resource management (CRM) and accident avoidance. Incidents usually don't happen because of one big foul-up. They generally are a result of numerous little things all going wrong, in perfect order, that lead to a catastrophe. We refer to it as Swiss cheese. Usually the holes in the Swiss cheese don't line up. You can't see through a hunk of Swiss cheese. Unless . . .

If you want to mix metaphors, it's a perfect storm. The pilot didn't sleep, or got in a fight with his wife, the crewmember didn't do a full walk-around, or was on their phone during take-off, the mechanic left a switch toggled on instead of off, or there was an imperfect design by an engineer a long time ago. Each of these in itself wouldn't cause an accident. But all of them together can be deadly.

Every year our EMS pilots are required to do a check ride with an instructor pilot. Because we work as a team, the crew is also on board for the flight. The pilot is tested on their flight proficiency, and the crew is tested on CRM and pilot assistance. The flight lasts a little over an hour and is usually at night because the instructor needs to train and rate everyone in the use of NVGs (night-vision goggles).

The "highlight" of the training is autorotation testing. I was lucky because I was flying with Sam, a retired Army pilot. Sam is dialed.

An autorotation simulates power loss to the main rotor system. Your first thought is likely *Game over.* If the main rotor blades lose power, the helicopter is dropping out of the sky like a rock thrown off a cliff. But that is not entirely true.

A couple of things to point out: If the rotor blades lock up, stop spinning, say from the gearbox arresting, then yes, you do fall out of the sky like a rock from a cliff. But if you lose power and the blades keep spinning, there's a chance. The pilot has to do everything right, but, like Lloyd Christmas from *Dumb and Dumber*, I'm saying there's a chance.

There are three primary controls in the helicopter. They are not totally analogous to the controls in an airplane. I am a private pilot and most of my time is in a fixed-wing aircraft. I got my license prior to entering the Academy to improve my chances of acceptance. That's how I sold it to my parents when I started lessons at seventeen. But really I started training because I simply loved to fly.

During medical school, I started to dabble in flying a helicopter. I have about thirty hours of rotor time. That means I have attempted to fly a helicopter.

I'll say there is one major difference between a helicopter and an airplane: an airplane *wants* to fly, and a helicopter, most decidedly, does not. The first time I flew in a helicopter I probably was a bit cocky. I had already had my pilot's license for some time. I strapped in for my first lesson and thought that I would be a natural.

The instructor explained the three major controls. The first is the cyclic. This joystick is held in the pilot's right hand, and in bigger helicopters, it comes out of the floor between the pilot's legs. It controls the pitch and bank of the aircraft. The cyclic allows you to move forward, backward, and sideways in a helicopter. The second controls are the antitorque pedals. They help manipulate the yaw, or twisting, of the aircraft. Finally, there is the collective (which includes the throttle). The collective is located down and to the left of the pilot's seat and is held in the left hand. It moves up and down, controlling the helicopter's altitude. Additionally, there is a twist grip on the collective that allows the pilot to control the throttle.

As we were ready to take off, the instructor told me to only worry about the cyclic. He told me to take my feet off the pedals and my hand off the collective. I was a little put off. I felt he was clearly underestimating my ability to fly.

Moments after lifting, he said, "Your helicopter."

He was indicating that I had control of the cyclic. Immediately, the helicopter began to shift back and forth. The oscillations became bigger and more pronounced. Similar to when you start to get speed wobbles on a bike or a skateboard. Every attempt at trying to bring things back in control only resulted in a more aggressive movement in the opposite direction. Like the frequency building on the previous wave in perfect harmony, we soon were careening out of control. I felt like the Tacoma Narrows Bridge in a windstorm. I was scared shitless. My mind was screaming, *Take the stick! Take the stick!*

But I couldn't get the words out of my mouth because I was too busy peeing my pants. I was completely overwhelmed, and we were on the brink of crashing. Just when I thought it was too late, the instructor took over control of the helicopter. He quickly and effortlessly settled the movement to a hover. I was breathing like a fat kid running up a flight of stairs. Again, a little mean-spirited, I know. But I thought it. Sorry.

"OK," he said calmly. "Nice one."

I didn't respond.

He added, "Don't overcorrect. More finesse."

Yeah, Captain Obvious, I needed a lot more finesse.

Sam, our pilot for this check ride, always used finesse. As I said, he is dialed. Toward the end of the check ride it was time to practice the autorotation. Angela, my crewmate, a flight nurse, hates autorotations. She became tense even before we started the maneuver.

Flying over the open field next to the airport, the instructor suddenly pulled the power off. The helicopter lurched as we began to drop out of the sky. My stomach went up into my throat and Angela let out a yelp, and she grabbed the seat and my leg. Sam went to work. By adjusting the collective, Sam kept us in the sweet spot. As the ground rapidly approached, Sam called out the altitude to the instructor. Although we were "gliding," our decent was fast nonetheless. If Sam didn't do anything, we would crash hard.

Just before that happened, Sam changed the pitch, or the angle of attack, of the rotor blades. The blades began to bite into the air. The kinetic energy from the spin was converted to lift, and the descent slowed. In fact, the helicopter flared just before hitting the ground. We came in for a soft landing. Definition of *finesse*.

Pat Mahany died on July 3, 2015, in a HEMS-related helicopter crash. He had been an EMS pilot for twenty-seven years. He was a cowboy with a big mustache, the kind you'd expect from an aging frontiersman or a grizzled Vietnam pilot. According to a profile in *Autorotate*, a magazine about helicopter pilots, Mahany "wears a larger-than-life, hard-chargin' Irishman veneer thinly draped over a big, soft heart of gold." He rescued countless people and saved countless lives through his work. It was in his nature, his DNA.

In Vietnam, Pat flew 1,200 combat hours and was shot down three times. He had been awarded a Bronze Star and Purple Heart.

I found this online:

> *Last August I was airlifted conscious, but in critical condition, from Vail Valley Med Center to Denver. I was vacationing with my husband and 3 kids from Minneapolis, MN when I started to have internal bleeding. When I was told in the Vail ER that I would have to go to Denver via helicopter I began to panic. I am afraid of heights and*

flying in a big plane makes me nervous, how was I going to stay calm in a little helicopter? Shortly thereafter, two men in flight suits entered the ER and introduced themselves as Matt and Dave. They took me via ambulance to the helicopter pad. As they loaded me into the helicopter I made eye contact with the pilot. He had a mustache and friendly eyes as I like to describe them. He looked to be about my dad's age and I wanted to ask him if he flew in Vietnam (my dad flew in a Huey helicopter in Vietnam from '67-'68 as the mechanic) but the mood was all business between the pilot, Matt and Dave, so I decided to wait and ask at a later time. I instantly felt at ease with MY pilot. He had a calm, strong, assured presence. Did I mention friendly eyes. As we took off in the early morning it was just light enough for me to see the mountains around us. I looked out to find the Gore Range when I realized it was right in front of us. I was in AWE of the gorgeous scene. We flew right OVER it, actually through two peaks of it. Here I was in critical condition having an unforgettable awesome experience. I immediately thought, "wow my pilot has a fantastic view out his office window." We had to land quick in Frisco to pick up more blood for me and then we took off for Denver. It was a crystal clear morning and we got to see the sun rise as *we flew east. It was absolutely beautiful!! We landed in Denver and they pulled me out of the helicopter so fast I didn't get a chance to say anything let alone thank my pilot. I vowed I would find him, along with Matt and Dave, as soon as I got through my crisis and back to MN. I searched in vain last August. I figured once the bill came I could track them all. It was billed through the hospital and listed as air ambulance so my search lead nowhere. Last Friday there was a quick story on our local news stating a medical helicopter crashed west of Denver. I had a sinking feeling as I looked it up online. When I saw the photo of Patrick I burst into tears. I'm so very sorry I never got the chance to thank him for saving my life and giving me my first and BEST helicopter ride ever!! I was so scared and nervous and he made me feel comforted without saying a word. I wish I had been able to ask him about Vietnam and thank him for his service to our country. I'm so very sorry for your loss and the pain you, as his family, are going through. My hope is that my story comforts you some, as it reminds you of his spirit, his presence, his service to many, and his happy eyes and mustache. He is forever in my heart as one of my angels. May God bless and comfort you all at this very difficult time.*

—Cari Girk

Pat had let the flight program know that he was retiring in the fall. After all the years of service and flying he had decided to step back, take a breather. He was a Coloradan and loved all the things the state has to offer—hiking, fishing, skiing. He always loved fast cars.

Pat was a staunch Catholic, the Irish kind that cracks jokes, says inappropriate things, gets into trouble, but always shows up to Mass with the utmost respect for God and the clergy.

Now unexpectedly, all of us were at this funeral. And Catholics don't do *just* funerals. This was going to be a Mass.

The bagpipers marched out and everyone sat.

CHURCH

"Blue on Black" Kenny Wayne Shepherd

I went to Catholic high school. Not because we were Catholic, but because it was a good and disciplined education. As a result, I learned the logistics of Mass: when to stand, when to kneel, what to say, and so on. It still comes in handy when I go to Catholic ceremonies, like weddings and funerals.

I was raised Lutheran. I think it was because my family is from Denmark. A ton of Danes are Lutherans, or so I'm told.

I don't totally know the history, but I know there was some big rift when my parents got married. My dad was a Catholic, and my mom a Lutheran. Like a good husband, he was going to "convert." They said things like that because switching from Catholic to Lutheran back in the day was a big deal. Just ask Luther. My dad's family almost disowned him. It wasn't like he was going on jihad or anything, but I guess it was pretty dramatic.

We were regulars, every Sunday. It was a "family day"—church, then some activity with the family. I wanted to do normal kid stuff, hang out with my friends, or go to the creek, swim, anything that didn't involve church.

Lutheran churches are a bit boring. I don't know if you've been. Turns out there are two types of Lutheran churches, and yes, in my opinion, both are boring. One stricter, and the other more laid back. I was raised in the "laid back" version. Way more chill than a Catholic service, but way less cool than the current church I go to, with a rock band and a tattooed pastor.

There always seemed to be some drama growing up in that boring church. One of the pastors, an awesome figure in my memory and an Air Force general, died of cancer. I really liked him. Another guy, who took over later, had an affair with one of the married women of the congregation. Real drama around that. I think he ended up being a computer salesman or something. Then there were the typical small-world political battles and cliques, just like anywhere.

I was never too impressed with church as a kid. I definitely didn't go to figure out the world. I went, first, because my parents made me, and second, it seemed we, as a family, went because that is just what you were supposed to do.

I don't recall having a real sense of figuring out the tough predicaments, the real-life issues like bullies, cancer, babies dying, divorce, and genocide. We never addressed a kid coming into the ER and not going home, or a rescue pilot dying in a fiery crash, or a pastor sleeping with a parishioner. That, I was left to deal with on my own. Which, as a young boy and much into my later life, meant I didn't. I had better things to do.

There was a comedian named Mitch Hedberg. He has a joke that reminds me of church.

"I have a shirt that says Dry Clean Only." A pause to let the crowd try to figure out where he was going. "Do you know what that means?" Again, a pause as the audience contemplates the answer. "It means it's dirty."

If it was too much trouble, I probably wasn't addressing it.

This became clearer years later when I returned home for Christmas, a grown man with a family of my own. My sister was there as well, sitting next to me as usual, harassing me, but not letting my parents see. Some things never change. The pastor started his sermon in his long, slow, singsong delivery. Same pastor that was there when I was younger. Not the computer salesguy but the next guy. I do a heck of an impression. If only there was a way to convey it in a book. His message was about Clarence, his cat.

> *"I remember riding home from church on Christmas Eve, lost in the big back seat of the Vista Cruiser, with blue paint and fake wood paneling running up the side, tires nearly worn out from driving all us kids to and from school, upholstery worn from our active imaginations and games in the back, while my father tried to ignore our noise. We were un-seat-belted, as usual, fighting with one another, clearly from the excitement of Christmas Eve. . . ."*

This description would go on and on for another five minutes, still slow, clear, and melodic.

". . . Clarence was waiting at home. He had the attitude that he just didn't care, as he licked his paws one by one, first the left, then the right. He placed his paws down, only to be reminded that he hadn't done a good enough job and lifted his left foot again. When finally finished, he meandered over to the presents, the way cats do, in his self-absorbed, unbothered way, unaware of the excitement that was pent up in all of us. . . ."

More description about Clarence—like a molasses-and-double-chocolate s'more metaphor cake. He gave a pause to push up his spectacles.

". . . The table was decorated with a doily from my grandmother, who used to rock in her chair, smiling at us as we fought over the coconut-covered cookies. . . ."

Still more description about the table and again Clarence. I hope you're getting the point. I can hand you my dull pencil for your eye if you're ready.

I looked over at my sister, who had the same look on her face. This was church. The church that we grew up in, with stories of Clarence and a Vista Cruiser. There was no substance. Just filler, fluff. I wanted the meat lover's pizza with everything, but it wasn't served at my church.

I can tell you a lot more about the pastor's cat and his childhood Christmas Eve. What I can't tell you is the point of Clarence the cat. I honestly don't remember. I don't think it moved me nearly as much as the diarrhea of color commentary.

While we sat there and listened to the sermon and the story of the cat, I had a realization: this is what I had grown up with in church, and that's why I didn't want to go. Now older, sitting next to my sister and listening, I realized this didn't have much to do with my regular life.

Like most people, I find that a funeral makes me reflect. I can't help but think about my own life and my own family as I watch the ceremony unfold. What if that were me? What if I died tomorrow? What if something happened to my family? Why this? Why that? What is the point? All of these feelings and questions stirred up in me.

I'm a spiritual person. Even with the Lutheran church thing. And even with the Catholic high school thing. My belief grew from my personal quest and search. Not church and certainly not Catholic school. It came from what I perceive is real and true.

I see God in everything. And this is why I spend so much time so vexed. This is why God pisses me off. As I sat in the amphitheater at the funeral that day, looking out at the beautiful lake and the jagged mountains, I couldn't help but be in awe of the beauty, the creation of it all. But if I just changed my view slightly, tilted my head downward a bit, looked left toward the stage, I saw a dead pilot and a substitute immaculate helmet. I saw his family mourning the loss of a husband, father, grandfather, and friend.

These two perceptions, views really, are at odds with one another. I'm told God is beautiful and magnificent and awesome, kittens and Clarence. But at the same time, this omniscient, omnipotent God also is the orchestrator of pain, suffering, and sadness. It has to be Him, if He is all-powerful, all-knowing, and created everything. That logic follows.

On the surface, I could just pass it off, say that it's evil in the world or that it's not of God, but I can't do that. My wife and I get into these "discussions" all the time. She is a wonderful soul; I love her to death. I'll get into that in a bit. She was raised in a religious family and spent some of her earlier years leading youth groups. That's why she speaks Spanish, because she spent considerable time in Costa Rica doing mission work. Like so many people, she feels that if she questions these confusing things, she is losing faith. These questions don't have an easy answer and likely don't have an answer at all. That's why, she says, you must have faith. She tells me to have more faith.

But that isn't a solution, not for me. And I don't believe lack of faith is my problem. Well . . . it isn't my primary problem.

Our existence is hidden, veiled behind only part of the picture that I may never fully see, but to me, that doesn't mean I stop looking, questioning, driving toward an explanation. Maybe it's the scientist in me. I can't let it go. The search, or the desire to search and understand, doesn't imply a lack of faith.

If there is a wizard behind the curtain, then I want to find him, even if it is a sham, a great Oz pulling levers and blowing smoke screens. I search and struggle and delve deep into thoughts and feelings because I want to know. I need to know if this makes any sense. At times like the funeral, sitting in the amphitheater looking at a gorgeous view and the results of a terrible accident, I need to know that I'm not just an insignificant collection of atoms to be tortured by the whim of electrical charge.

My anger, annoyance, and frustration with God might feel wrong, especially because I went to Catholic school, but how else should I feel? I was trained growing up to trust God, not to question, to stay on the straight and narrow. Lutheran church–style.

That doesn't work for me . . . at all. Why would I have this personality that lets me delve into science and medicine, that questions all the cool things I see around me, only to have it shut down by the most profound questions of our existence?

This place, our universe, isn't just thrown together, willy-nilly, like some mad scientist doing an experiment that makes no sense. There are rules. It's a puzzle, beautifully constructed to give us purpose and meaning.

If I wasn't a doctor, I think I would have been a physicist. I might not have been smart enough, but I think I would have tried. My dad used to tell me, "Son, I was too smart to be an economist, not smart enough to be a physicist, so I became a mathematician." He is aware that I graduated with a degree in economics, but that is beside the point.

But this is why I bring up physics. Because it's hard, and interesting, and puzzling. My son is currently taking physics in college as an engineering student. He summed it up a different way: "Physics is dumb." He sent a picture of a page of math homework handwritten in his notebook. It looked quite complicated, but also nicely choreographed over the entire landscape of his page. The caption on the WhatsApp picture said, "To be honest, I don't even know what I'm doing here."

And that is exactly what I'm talking about.

There's no way that physics—so magnificent, confusing, and awe inspiring—follows a set of rules, while at the same time, the emotional and spiritual part of this world is just an afterthought, with no rhyme or reason. That would be so . . . inelegant. And I don't see the world as inelegant. Physics isn't the problem. It's my understanding of physics that troubles me. What I'm trying to say about the spiritual part is that the problem is with me. I just can't see it or figure it out.

All that we experience allows us to grow and feel and see, if only in glimpses, the deep, unexplainable truth. We might not find all the answers, but that's part of the master plan, just like physics. Frustrating for sure, like my son's homework, but still part of the plan.

This leads me back to faith. These questions and working through the confusion are my way to faith. I'm exploring because I have faith, at least enough to get started, and that's really all anyone needs. A small match to light a fire.

So, I disagree with my wife. A risky position to take. True, we all need to have more faith, but, fundamentally, I don't think lack of faith is my problem. My faith forces me to spend my time and brainpower trying to address what I see, feel, and experience. I don't like to accept the answer "You just need to have more faith." I know I have faith. That's why I'm sitting here writing.

For me to understand all this, to even scratch the surface of this, I didn't need more church. I needed more life. I needed my patients, the real-life experiences and observations of people living in incredibly raw moments. I needed the white coat. I needed to be what Arnold P. Gold wanted me to be. I needed kids and pilots dying. I needed cancer patients and gunshot wounds.

That sounds awful. But what I'm trying to say is that I need to look at the things that happen in actual life. I need to accept the dirty dry cleaning. My life, right here and now, without any kind of filter. I need the gritty and dirty images, the kind that make me cringe and close my eyes. Even the emotions that try to pull me into the abyss. I need it all, every breath, every dance, every death. Everything. Uncensored.

GREEN MONSTER

"I'll Find You" Lecrae ft. Tori Kelly

The turbine started with a deep whine, and the smell of Jet A fuel spread across the roof of the hospital. The Green Monster—that's the nickname for our green and blue jet-ranger helicopter—came to life as it sat against the backdrop of the Rocky Mountains. I caught the pilot's eye through the windshield as I walked toward him and broke into a Gene Wilder/Richard Pryor *That's right, we bad* strut. He started to laugh and deliberately nodded his head slowly up and down as he pushed his bottom lip. He was consenting to the "badness." I latched the clasp of my helmet chinstrap and bent over to pull the disconnect for the battery cable that fit into the nose of the chopper.

I climbed through the side door into my seat, buckling my harness. Underneath my tinted visor, I could see the rhythmic change of shadow to sun as the blades slowly started to spin. With a *cha-clunk*, the hatch latched into place, and I slid the window open to feel the cool air. I plugged in my headset. "Tst, Tst." I hissed with my tongue against my teeth so I could hear myself for a radio check.

"You're good," said the pilot. In the background, ATIS, the automated weather report, gave its standard flight info: *This is information Juliet. 1835 Zulu weather. Set altimeter 12239. . . .*

I arranged the medical bag in front of me on the floor. Space is at a premium in the Bell 407. *The sports car of medical helicopters,* the pilot would say. Fun to fly, but not a lot of luxury. My partner, Linda, was situated on her side of the cabin. She smiled at me as I made a face while trying to pull down my flight suit by the thighs. Any guys out there who wear flight suits know what I'm talking about. They always ride up into your crotch, and I was having a little "situation."

"AirLife 1, lifting off Denver Downtown. Departure to the southwest," the pilot said in his formal military tone. Pilots always have that supersmooth voice, like they're on tranquilizers or something. Even when things are going poorly, they always sound so nonchalant. I was on a commercial airline once. We were coming in for a landing in foul weather, and the approach seemed aggressively prolonged. Then suddenly, full power, and the jumbo jet started to lurch upward at a steep angle of attack. I sank back in my seat. We were going to die. I was sure of it.

After a ridiculously long silence, the pilot came over the intercom. "Ahhhhh, we are going to go around. The weather was worse than reported." He continued, as if he was ordering a soft drink at a drive-through. "It's not like we didn't plan for this. We'll have enough fuel, no problem." The first thing I want to point out is that he said it slow and deep. Calm. The second thing is, Why the hell is he mentioning the fuel? Is he watching the gauge pin itself on Empty or what? I mean, why even mention it? Again, I digress. But the point is, pilots always sound so calm. Like they have ice blood or something.

I looked out the window of the helicopter and saw one of the other flight nurses who was not flying today, standing off to the side. She gave me a short salute, and I returned my standard hang-loose sign. I checked my side for obstacles and obstructions. The pilot said, "Coming up." We hovered for a moment. "Power is good." And then we were off. The car crash was twenty minutes out.

This was the perfect job for me. I'm sure the flight thing was left over from the Air Force Academy and my childhood. Aside from having to wear a corny blue suit with a reflective stripe down the leg, or lamenting the possibility of crashing, the job had very little downside. I struggled when I left the Academy. I tried to run away from flying because it hurt. But ultimately, I love it, and I never predicted how I would be pulled back to the sky. There is nothing more invigorating than flying over a city in a helicopter, taking care of a really sick patient. It amazes me, all the pieces of the puzzle that had to fall into place to make this happen. Without the Air Force Academy, without my roommates, and so many little things, I would never be here. And I love being here.

As a resident, I worked as the liaison for Stanford's Life Flight program. On my first flight, I had been so clueless. I had tried to play it chill, but I'm sure I looked like a tool. I think I missed a central line. I'm not saying that I don't miss anymore, but I just seemed extra-lame.

I felt the power surge, and the rotor blades gripped the air. We gained altitude. It happens so effortlessly. The physics of it still baffle me. And I say that having studied the physics of it. It was a beautiful day, and the view was unbelievable. Flying in a helicopter over Denver, or any city, is fantastic. You're close enough to almost reach out and touch the buildings and people, yet far enough away to be in your own cocoon.

My pilot, Jesse, is an ex-special forces military man. I'm sure he's flown into some nasty situations, which gives me confidence when I'm riding in the back of his helicopter. He would joke that he could land our 407 anywhere in this job because he had as much time as he needed with no one shooting at him.

I first got to know Jesse just a month into the job. We were at a conference in Texas. My company had taken our helicopter to show off the new medical interior system in the exhibit hall. At the end of the conference, they disassembled the rotors so the helicopter could fit through the conference center doors. It was wheeled into the middle of a central hotel courtyard. We stood and watched as our mechanic reassembled the rotor blades. Twisting a slightly oversized torque wrench, he straddled the blade on top of the engine canopy. No real strain or effort. That was it. A couple of bolts, a big wrench, and we were good to go. I looked up and saw the hotel extend upward about four stories on all sides of the courtyard. We were going to launch straight up—totally ballistic. Maverick- and Goose-style.

As we buckled our seatbelts, I asked Jesse about the rotors. I was curious as to the likelihood of the things flying off once he put in the power. Seemed like a reasonable question, considering I just had watched the mechanic hand-wrench them on. I barely knew Jesse, and he answered totally straight-faced. "I don't worry about that. Neither should you. If they come off, there's nothing either of us can do." He paused, flicking some switches, going through his checklist. "We'd be dead." He paused again. I didn't say anything. I just looked out the front window at the people watching. He added, "Dead, dead."

Our mission today was up one of the canyons. In the mountains, we sometimes purposefully fly between the ridgelines, saving some altitude. We snaked up and approached the accident scene. As is customary, we circled around to get a good look at the situation, noting any obstacles or hazards that might try to jack us on landing or takeoff. The accident looked like a mess.

Two cars had creamed each other. A couple of fire trucks blocked traffic at either end. A hose line tracked across the street, and tools, the big ones—jaws of life— were laid out next to one of the cars. An additional fire truck sat just a bit south on the road. That was our target for landing.

"Engine 2501, this is Med Evac 1, how do you copy?" Doing her best pilot impression, the nurse kept her voice steady and assured.

"AirLife 1, Engine 2501. Copy loud and clear. Approach from the south and land just south of the engine. We have spotters. Obstacles include a fence to the east and a small ditch to the west of the highway. Winds from the north about ten miles per hour."

"Copy that."

Jesse completed one last circle and then came in from the south. People think we just rip into landing sites, but that's not the case. This is an extremely hazardous phase of flight. Jesse took his time, ensuring the blades had good bite and there wasn't anything we missed. "One hundred. Fifty. Twenty-five. Ten."

First the right skid, then immediately the left. There was a slight bounce as Jesse let the full weight of the system onto the landing gear. The rotor blades still spinning, I disconnected my mic jack, hopped out, and moved toward the accident through the mud and wet. The car had spun off the road after the impact. The medic gave us a brief, pressured report. He had to yell due to the rotor slap in the distance and the fact that I was still taking off my helmet.

The patient sounded bad. I moved to the car where the fire department was extricating. They just about had him out. The driver was a little younger than me. We could have been friends in a different scenario. As I continued to get a report, my partner moved to the patient and performed a brief exam. I quickly realized the paramedic was correct in his reported assessment. The patient was serious.

Fire got the patient onto a backboard as they pulled him from the car. We laid him on the ground so we could do another, more thorough, check before getting the heck out of Dodge.

ABCs. Practice how you play. Be consistent.

His airway was intact; he was able to talk to us. He had difficulty breathing and his respiratory rate was rapid—either from pain or chest pathology, no way to know just yet. His saturation was low: 78 percent. So, probably pathology.

My partner pointed out the crepitus on exam. Crepitus is a crackling and grating feeling under the skin, and in this situation likely represented a pneumothorax. A needle decompression was performed on the right. She had placed a large bore IV catheter through the wall of the anterior chest at the level of the second intercostal space (between the ribs). The intent is to relieve air from a pneumothorax (a "popped lung").

His abdomen was bruised from the seat belt sign across his waist, and he had mild bruising on both sides. It was firm, distended, and exquisitely tender. All bad signs. This guy had internal injuries. Nothing we could fix here. He needed a surgeon, stat. Our best treatment was going to be high speed fuel expenditure to the hospital.

Twenty things needed to be done at one time. I prioritized and tried to keep my impatience in check. Interventions, loading, liftoff—they all take too long.

As we cruised east, I took a brief look out the window and started to recognize the scenery. I could see the various freeway intersections coursing through the outskirts of Denver and knew that we were about ten minutes out. Just about that time, the patient started to go downhill. He was shivering and having more difficulty breathing. This was compounded by a drop in his pressure to 70/P. I reassessed and tried to coach him. My partner finished her radio report with "hot offload."

There are two types of patient transfer, "cold offload" and "hot offload." Hot offload meant that we were not going to take the time to shut the helicopter down prior to exiting. We'd disembark the patient with the rotor blades still spinning. It's a bit unnerving for the patient and staff at the hospital, but this guy was on his way to the dark side.

As the skids hit the roof, the patient looked up at me, and I tried to reassure him. "Almost there, man." He was mumbling something through his non-rebreather. I lifted it slightly off his face and bent over so I could hear through my helmet.

"Am I going to die?" he asked with wild eyes. He was serious. When a patient asks you that question, you should always take them seriously. That's from experience.

"Hang in there. We'll be in the ER in a sec," I answered. The truth was that I didn't know the answer to his question. I quickly disconnected the mounted monitor and equipment. I released the stretcher retention system as the flight nurse finished opening the bi-folding side door.

The staff met us with a gurney, and we slid the pram out of the helicopter. Riding the elevator down to the first floor, we tried to untangle and manage all the cords and IVs coming off the patient. As we entered the resuscitation room, we met the trauma surgeon and gave the report. I wiped the sweat off my forehead.

"Patient is a forty-year-old male involved in an MVC." (A motor vehicle collision.) "Prolonged extrication. Complaining of SOB and severe abdominal pain. Vitals initially stable except for a low sat at 78 percent. Decompressed on scene. He stabilized but en route pressure and stats started to drop. Exam showed increased work of breathing and tender and distended abdomen. Patient has two 16s in place. One liter of normal saline. We gave one hundred of fentanyl and four of Zofran."

"OK," he said as he moved toward the patient, patting me on the back as he squeezed by.

A resident perked his head up. "FAST is positive." FAST stands for Focused Assessment with Sonography in Trauma. The resident had quickly performed a bedside ultrasound that revealed free fluid in the abdomen. This likely represented blood.

Another resident began cutting into his chest with a scalpel to place a chest tube.

Within only a few moments, the trauma surgeon turned to walk out of the room. "We're going to the OR." The staff moved behind him, making it happen. The patient rolled by me and Linda. He still had the wide eyes. He clearly was having more difficulty breathing now. The elevator door shut, and the patient was gone.

NOT LIKE TV

"Lost Soul" Bruce Hornsby

It's not like it is on TV, watching someone die. *Grey's Anatomy* makes it all seem so cool and dramatic. Music playing in the background, pained facial expressions on good-looking actors. But when a patient really dies, when *my* patient dies, it isn't such great drama. It bites away a piece of my soul. Like a service charge for the job.

As a boy, I had a stuffed Bugs Bunny. It was one of the few times I won anything at an amusement park. By a pure fluke, I tossed a ping-pong ball that landed in the red box in a vast waffle board of mostly white boxes. I wasn't the stuffed animal type of kid, but you can't just disregard something that fortune set on your lap. Even though I preferred my action figures, skateboard, and BMX bike, Bugs had a special place. He would be my patient and I'd be his surgeon.

Unfortunately, Bugs was sickly. I'd have to operate on him every few weeks. I had acquired the tools, a pickup and a clamp, during a school tour at the hospital. I supplied the pocketknife. My mom would hide a marble somewhere in Bugs's body, and I'd then have to "diagnose" the problem and take him to the operating room. I became an expert surgeon. My incisions were perfect. My closures would have made the best seamstress raise an eyebrow and take note. I took it all very seriously. I mean, come on, these were very risky procedures I was performing, under less than ideal circumstances, on my desk, in my room, in questionably sterile conditions.

The most amazing aspect of all these surgeries was my success rate. Bugs's doctor never failed him, ever. In over twenty surgeries I never lost Bugs. It might have been touch and go at times, but in the end, he lived. He always lived.

It's weird for me, being with a dead person. I've seen a lot of them but never have gotten totally used to it. On the surface, sure, but not on the inside, deep down. They look like they're wearing makeup. Like powder and cover-up. The wrinkles, the small ones, that you don't worry about when living, often disappear. The muscle tension is gone, like a Botox treatment. The skin becomes flat, and the subtle shades of color leave.

My first dead person was my nana. She died from colon cancer when I was seven. I have only glimpses of memory: her white hair, her apron, a crooked nose. I really didn't know what cancer was at the time, but I knew it was bad. It made her skinny, pale, and bedridden. It also made her itch her nose all the time. In hindsight, that was from the morphine, but I associated it with the cancer. She wore a nasty bag that smelled foul and came out of her stomach. I knew I didn't want cancer.

The night before her funeral, we went to the mortuary to view her open casket. It was similar to being in church, but different. I felt as though I couldn't make a sound, like I'd better behave or there'd be bigger ramifications than a shushing from my parents. Her coffin had that fluffy, satin padding wrapped around the inside edges. It looked like if you dropped it, the body inside would remain protected and unbroken. Maybe coffins get dropped often, I don't know.

When we walked up, I just stared at her. It felt irreverent and respectful in the same moment. I tried to catch her moving, anything—a flinch, a small breath, or a little eye flutter—that would give her away, the same way they had always given me away when I was trying to trick my sister into believing that she had knocked me out. But as I looked, Nana didn't move. She was either a really good faker or really dead.

When I was younger I used to dream about the big save. I didn't always know that I wanted to be a doctor. I realize you might not believe me on that one because I used to operate on Bugs, but I'm telling the truth. It never crossed my mind. But the hero thing, that was legit. Fighter pilot legit. One day, I knew that the moment would arrive when all eyes would turn to me, and I'd step up to the plate. Just like Babe Ruth, I'd point to center field before the pitch and then belt it into the bleachers. I knew I wanted to hit the home run. I just didn't consider the fact that hitting a home run every now and then came with so many strikeouts.

In college, one of my worst classes was philosophy. We had an assignment that I thought was a complete waste of time. We were told a story and then had to write a paper in response. It went something like this:

> Amelia had a boat that she loved dearly. It was a beautiful, brand-new, red rowboat. Like a good owner, she registered the boat with the DMV, and named it *Sea Squirrel*. She was extravagantly meticulous in its care. Every time there was even the smallest flaw in the boat, she'd replace it. Whether that meant repainting it, replacing a board, or changing out the hardware, she'd do it. Everything that came off the boat she saved, in the far corner of the warehouse that housed the *Sea Squirrel*.
>
> Little did Amelia know that there was a secret *Sea Squirrel* admirer. Emma, another girl in town, loved the *Sea Squirrel*. In fact, she was obsessed. She wanted the *Sea Squirrel* to be her own. So every time Amelia replaced something on the boat and discarded the old piece onto the pile, Emma would scavenge it. Eventually, over the years, Emma had scavenged everything original. She put the whole thing back together, recreating the original *Sea Squirrel*. She went to the DMV to register it.
>
> Well, this caused quite a ruckus. Neither Amelia nor Emma wanted to yield

her position as the true owner of the *Sea Squirrel.*

"Now, your assignment is to write a detailed paper proving whether Amelia or Emma is the true owner of the *Sea Squirrel.*"

That was the assignment. Huh? Straight up busy work. A complete waste of time. But, hey, premed. I needed to get an A. I was driven and determined. I sat in the library and thought hard about the question. There had to be a correct answer. There had to be an answer that would get me a good grade.

There's not. There's not a right answer. This caused me some angst. You could get a good grade no matter who you chose as the boat's rightful owner. You just had to give a convincing argument.

I think about that class frequently. Way more than I think about my differential equations class. It's because it didn't have a right answer. In school, in work, and in life, I want an answer. I want to know how to make it work out in my favor. I want to have the control of knowing that if I stick to a particular path I will get the outcome I desire. But man, life just isn't like that. It's a quandary, a confusing riddle. Even worse, a riddle for which I have no idea of the solution. To be honest, sometimes I don't even get the question.

In college, I never stomached another philosophy class. I just couldn't bear it.

THE MATRIX

"So What'cha Want" Beastie Boys

The *Matrix* is a great movie. It combined an ingenious plot with nonstop action and amazing special effects. Like most guys my age, I thought it was right up my alley. If you haven't seen it, see it, but let me give a brief recap. If you have, just bear with me for a sec.

In the movie, sentient machines hold humans in a virtual reality prison, the Matrix. The humans don't even know they are in prison. The machines control every facet of perceived existence within the Matrix to pacify humans, using them to generate energy for their ongoing survival. The movie's plot revolves around a few humans who have escaped from the Matrix to see the truth: machines control and harvest humans.

There's a scene when one of the leading characters, Neo, is offered "freedom" from the Matrix into true reality. Morpheus, the leader of a band of "enlightened" humans holds his hand out in front of Neo. In it are two pills, one red and one blue. He tells Neo, "You take the blue pill, the story ends. You wake up in your bed and believe whatever you want to believe. You take the red pill. You stay in Wonderland, and I show you how deep the rabbit hole goes."

Wanting to know the truth, he takes the red pill.

Neo becomes "unplugged." He awakens to the grungy, cold, and stark reality outside the Matrix. He's enlightened, but with it comes hardship and pain. Before he took the pill he lived a normal life as a computer programmer inside the virtual reality of the Matrix. Now he fights for mankind's existence in the austere environment of the "real" world.

As the plot unfolds, Neo's disgruntled crewmate, Cypher, laments that he should never have taken the damn red pill. "I know what you're thinking, 'cause right now I'm thinking the same thing. Actually, I've been thinking it ever since I got here: Why oh why didn't I take the *blue* pill?"

A couple of days after the flight, I checked in on the patient. He was living, but barely. They thought he would recover. Over the course of the conversation I found out that the patient had run out to get some Chinese takeout. He was almost home when he crashed. I've read the stats that accidents most often occur close to home. I think that's a probability thing—you're just close to home more often. It isn't like your neighborhood is a death trap or anything.

During the flight the patient had repeatedly told me he didn't know what happened. He never saw the other car. Never saw it coming.

There was a picture on the internet that went viral not too long ago. A photographer had caught a shot of a doctor in scrubs and a white coat, crunched down with one hand on a wall and the other on his face. The picture was taken after he had just lost a patient who had arrested. He clearly was shaken and had availed himself of a quiet moment outside by himself.

The reason the image went viral was because it showed compassion, feeling, and the emotions of a doctor. People, seeing the picture, were not only moved but surprised. Moved for obvious reasons, but surprised because the doctor was showing such despondence and pain.

This shouldn't be surprising. Doctors are affected. It's hard to be around death. It's hard to be around the uncertainty, the randomness, and the reality that anything can happen on any given day. And once it happens, there's the magnitude of loss and devastation that follows.

There are ramifications to bad things happening. Everything can change so suddenly, literally in a heartbeat. It applies to everyone. No one is immune. It doesn't matter who you are, what you've done, or what you plan to do in the future. And this nasty shit happens all . . . the . . . time.

I think about Pat. He'd flown hundreds—thousands—of missions. He was well respected and trusted. He was planning his retirement. Then, suddenly, wham, everything changes. Not just for Pat, but for his wife, his kids, their kids, his friends and coworkers. The ripple effect is less like a ripple and more like a tsunami.

Never saw it coming.

This brings me back to God.

It brings me back to who owned the dang *Sea Squirrel*.

I want answers. But there aren't any.

Why does this stuff happen?

I don't mean it simply, like *Why is it painful when a husband, father, or son dies?* It's obviously painful because we feel a loss. It hurts to realize we won't get to hear any more jokes, feel a strong embrace, or watch him rile the priest. We lose the future experience with the person.

I mean the *why* on a more philosophical level. It's a *Sea Squirrel* question. Why did Pat have to die? And hey, I get it. We are flesh and bone. We have to die at some point. It's the circle of life. Hakuna matata.

But I still can't help myself. I still want the *why*. And I don't even know totally what that means. And as I sit here writing, it's hard to even form the question. Do I mean, *Why does it have to happen?* I know everyone dies, so it doesn't quite catch the essence. Maybe I mean *Why does it happen suddenly? Why is it unexpected?* Or even better, *Why is it painful? Why did they suffer?*

My wife lost her father to leukemia. He was young and previously healthy. It's clear this doesn't make any sense to her. The same way it doesn't make sense that I had to do CPR on a friend of mine. It just is.

I'm not alone here. The *whys*, they quickly blow up in my face. There is a lot of badness out there. Not just trauma, but cancer. ISIS, suicide bombers, famine, genocide, suicide. The list goes on and on. It is inescapable. Not just for me but for everyone. Mainly because we have nonstop access to the internet.

Really, what I think it comes down to is simple and selfish. I'm wondering about my own personal *why*. *Why doesn't it happen on my terms?*

Back to the circle of life. People are going to die, because everyone does. OK. But what I want is for them to die when I want them to die. And how I want them to die. Which is never. And not badly. So wait. . . .

I sense a philosophy class calling my name.

To keep from being completely overwhelmed, I have to stop myself when things start to spiral out of control. I just stop. Not with the answer, but with a slightly different question. *What is my why?*

Let me step aside for a second. I have to apologize. This may not be the book you're looking for. I'll repeat. This may not be the book you're looking for. Because I don't have the answer.

I do have an observation. And that is why I just stop. I breathe. In and out. Breathe in, breathe out. Big forward, small back.

My observation is this.

I really, really love my kids. "I'm pretty into my wife" is an understatement. I love big complicated things like black holes and time. But I also love simple things. Like a sunrise. Like a smile. The moon is phenomenal. And it comes out all the time. Sometimes it even gets eclipsed. Phenomenal.

I enjoy how connected I can feel to the things that matter. I like that I can go to a school talent show and totally lose myself when my son gets on stage. Or I can hear my wife breathe in bed when she rolls over. Date nights at a good restaurant are up there. I'm fortunate to have friends.

So, that makes me think about how I got to these feelings. How I feel so connected.

How do I get to *my* why?

All of these images of awe and emotion, they didn't just appear out of nowhere. They didn't come for free.

The cost was my opening up, allowing myself the risk. The risk is what sets the stage, and without it I have nothing.

What is my risk? Losing someone I love, something I cherish. Suffering. Feeling emptiness. Squatting down beside a wall outside of the ER in the middle of the night when I think no one is looking. The risk is living life, and that life is going to fill the whole gamut of experience—both good and bad. I don't get one without the other. God knows that. He also knows that I won't always see it or know it. That sometimes I'm going to be really hurt and pissed off.

So, all this takes me back to *The Matrix*. Would I take the blue pill or the red pill?

Each and every time I try to work through a quagmire, I find myself a little deeper down the real-life rabbit hole. I think of it as a God rabbit hole, courtesy of the Wachowskis.

And that's exactly where I want to be.

So hell yeah, I'm taking the red pill.

I'm like Neo. I would take the red pill all over again, even with all I know, even with the loss of innocence, as predicted. Life is hard. But the more I experience, both good and bad, the more I'm amazed. It's like one opens up the other and vice versa. I cannot even imagine what is in store for me. My future is terrifying and exhilarating all at the same time. It's like a black hole singularity—simple, complex, confusing, fascinating. It's all my emotions, connections, and experiences threaded together to allow each additional moment in time. It's mind-numbing, and I mean that in an absolutely positive way.

Maybe the red pill isn't for everyone because it isn't always pleasant, but the journey and the struggle to look for the truth and meaning is what forces me to grow and lets me love. It lets me hope.

The red pill is a leap of faith. I recently went hang gliding in Brazil. As you prepare to launch off the platform, the instructor reminds you to run, sprint really, with confidence. If you hesitate, you won't have lift. Obviously I want some lift. So when he says go, I run like I mean it. Like I'm taking the red pill. And it is unbelievably exhilarating.

Like the doctor on the internet, I feel. I'm not immune to this stuff. And I don't want to be immune. I was trained to be calm under pressure. Like a warrior in battle. But that doesn't mean I don't feel. I used to struggle when I came home after a bad call or case. I would be ashamed that I hadn't shown emotion in the moment. Like I was some sort of ruthless robot. The family of the patient may have even thought I was cold and uncaring.

I want them to know that I wasn't. It was just a defense mechanism. It allowed me to do my job. But there is more to it than that. It allowed me to be human. I could not see horrific and disgusting things without totally being drawn in by the inevitable pull of a black hole. My defense *let* me take it in, just not all at once.

I want the red pill. I want to see it all. That means that being in the middle of the shitstorm is sometimes exactly where I need to be.

I don't know if you remember earlier in the book when I talked about the White Coat Ceremony. I quoted a passage from the Arnold P. Gold Foundation. When I graduated from Columbia, I was honored to win an award from the foundation. It is given to the student showing clinical excellence and humanism to their patients. At the time, I didn't truly understand the award. To me it seemed like somehow I had committed a con or scam. Tricked everyone into seeing the doctor I hoped to be. Not the doctor I was. I mentioned that I felt ashamed because I could control my emotions and focus on the patient, like a problem. But it turns out that it is necessary. It's necessary because I *am* human, because I can and do feel. There is no way to feel the gravity of a situation in the moment and not totally collapse in despair. That is the skill of a good ER doctor. Perform in the moment, reflect over a lifetime.

If all of this doesn't sound like a superhero manifesto, I'm sorry. Sure, I wanted to be a superhero, but through experience I've realized that doctoring is different. It's better because it is painful. And it doesn't always end like the movies.

Humanism. It means I am *trying* to understand. I'm certainly not there, and I probably never will be. Because that's life. It's a work in progress. I can be calm, steady, solid, because that's how I was trained. It is a tool. It allows me to finally man up and look in the eyes of a mother who has just lost her son. It allows me to admit that I don't know if a patient is going to live or die.

The red pill has allowed me to be caring but at the same time cold. It's the rabbit hole. Something I didn't understand before I jumped.

In *The Matrix Reloaded*, the Merovingian says, "Where some see coincidence, I see consequence. Where others see chance, I see cost." There is a cost to caring for dying people, suffering people. There is also a cost to knowing and loving my wife. There is a big cost to being so head over heels for my kids. And there is a consequence to everything in between.

I think a lot of us have a moment in our life, a metaphorical one, where we are offered the red pill or the blue pill. If we take the blue pill, we can keep everything status quo, floating on the surface without ever diving deep. Life as usual, steering clear of anything that offsets the balance. But if we decide to delve deeper, know the truth, if we take the red pill, a whole new world opens up, revealing everything worth caring about.

Maybe God is onto something. Maybe I need to give God a break. Perhaps when God is really pissing me off, he's trying to get my attention.

Dr. Morgan knew this when I sat in the White Coat Ceremony. Plenty of people are happy without ever stepping into the fray. Dr. Morgan wanted to make sure I wasn't one of them.

I had dreamed of being a fighter pilot but ended up a doctor. I pulled on my clean, crisp white coat, sitting there in that auditorium, thinking I knew what to expect. I had no idea. Dr. Morgan knew that hovering around death is like hovering around a black hole. Sometimes you can't escape. It draws you in, too far if you let it. At times it asks too much, like gravity relentlessly pulling away every photon of light.

But, if you can manage it, the event horizon opens everything. Right there on the cusp. Devastation or exhilaration. You need to tiptoe on the edge of despair to know life. The fear and loss opens up joy and amazement. It's like one leads to the other. Let me rephrase that: one allows the other.

I picked up my kids from school and drove them home. We talked about the day, tests, girlfriends, a fire drill. As usual, the dogs were ecstatic to see us. I threw the ball outside for a bit. I kissed my wife.

We had forgotten to thaw the meat so we decided to grab some Chipotle. It's only a mile down the road. The dogs jumped in the back of the truck, I flipped up the tailgate, and climbed into the cab.

As I turned the key, I paused. I looked at my hands. Nothing had changed. They were quiet. I thought about my flight. I remembered all the medicine, the physiology. I remembered the scene. Details. The smell of Jet A fuel, car oil, and water on pavement and mud. A ripped pocket from his pants. A leaky fire hose and the handlebar mustache on the firefighter. It was all so vivid. I remembered my patient's wild eyes. I remembered his question.

I squeezed my grip and released. Then again. As my hand opened I just stared, lost in the mission. I became aware of the lines in my skin. There was a single solid horizontal line spanning my entire palm. No cutoffs or breaks. It's a fusion of my heart line and my head line. I've had palm-reading friends tell me this is a good trait. They call it a simian line. In medicine, when a baby is born with a single palmar crease—that's what I call it—doctors worry about genetic defects, like Down's syndrome. Palm readers think it's good, doctors think it's bad. I think it's just because I had my hand folded that way in utero.

I put the truck in reverse and started to back out of the driveway.

Takeout, I thought.

Deadly.

PART IV

0.2 SECONDS

"Dream On" Aerosmith

I t was a beautiful day. A lot like today at Lake Dillon. Sun shining, beautiful sky with scattered clouds. No one expected anything bad to happen. No one ever does. They were going on a routine PR mission. They weren't picking up a patient. They were going to provide community education and outreach. It's a normal occurrence for flight programs. The helicopter crew needs to interact with ground EMS during patient exchanges. Everyone needs to be on the same page, hence the training and the PR.

Pat Mahany and his crew, Dave and Matt, did their standard preflight. Everyone walked around the helicopter to ensure nothing was out of place. Pat began his preflight checklist while Dave and Matt strapped themselves into their seats in the aft compartment.

The A Star, also known as the H125, is a single-engine jet turbine helicopter. It is a highly functional and frequently utilized helicopter. It's famous because it made a landing on Everest. It was a light and stripped-down version of the

AStar, and the landing was more like a touch-and-go, but they counted it.

"Clear," he yelled out the window.

Start up clearance—received
Rotor—free
Area—clear
Starter—on
When Ng 10%—fuel flow lever forward
Ng—increase
Control T with fuel flow control—checked

Slowly the turbine engine came to life. First it sounded like a hum, but then the turbo kicked in, and a deep, guttural mechanical noise filled the space. The blades started to turn. Slowly at first, with a *swoosh, swoosh* each time they completed a revolution. Soon they were spinning too fast to see, and the noise deepened.

Pat finished the remainder of the checklist.

Engine oil pressure—green
Warning lights—all out, exc. HORN/PITOT
Fuel boost pump 1 + 2—test each pump, pressure,
　　and light
Gyros (Att ind./DG)—on

"RPMs 100%, in the green," Pat said through the mic. "You all good back there?" Pat asked the crew.

"Good to go," the response.

With a slight pull of the collective, the AStar started to lift off. The sound changed to a more pronounced hum, accompanied by a repetitive slap, as the blades started to grab the air.

However, as soon as the skids lifted, something went wrong. The helicopter began to spin counterclockwise. This was the result of the torque from the main rotor blade. It caused the fuselage of a helicopter to spin in the opposite direction of the spinning blades. My engineering son could probably work out the math for this phenomenon. Torque is precisely why helicopters have the rear blade at the end of the tail boom. It spins perpendicular to the main rotor. The antitorque pedals control the blade to keep the rotation null and the helicopter pointed in the desired direction.

As the AStar started to lift, there was naturally more torque due to the power. Pat expected the reaction to the action. He had lifted hundreds, thousands of times. But this was different. The helicopter didn't respond. More pedal. Still no response.

The helicopter lifted to one hundred feet, now spinning out of control.

The brain can do amazing computations. But this was too much. Pat began to apply opposite pedal, as he had trained to do, but the helicopter continued to spin. He tried to lower the collective to bring it back down, but the helicopter was spinning too fast. It would likely flip if he landed. Once again, he pulled in more collective and lifted. But this added power, which added to the spin. The AStar drifted off the centerline and moved out over the parking lot to the side of the landing pad.

Careening ever more out of control, Pat lowered the collective to decrease the rate of spin. In the corner of the parking lot there was a camper trailer parked. It was totally out of sight and mind, and as the helicopter lost altitude, it spun into the stationary object.

It was a profound and sudden impact. It occurred thirty-two seconds into the flight. The flight paramedic's seat was jarred loose by the crash. So was the fuel tank.

Three point seven seconds after impact, fuel leaked onto the ground.

Zero point two seconds later, fire erupted.

The AStar was equipped from the factory with a soft fuel tank. There was no reinforced metal container designed to withstand an impact from a crash. Not even as good as your Ford.

Heat, noise, pain. It all happened in a literal instant.

The paramedic unstrapped himself from the dislodged seat and attempted to escape. But only briefly. Seeing that Pat was strapped into his seat, he returned to try to save his friend. The flames overcame him.

The crash was cinematic and epic. Inside the hospital, the staff heard the explosion, and many scrambled outside to see what had happened. One of the CAT scan techs ran outside and saw the helicopter on fire. He quickly grabbed the fire extinguisher and was able to douse the flames enough to pull Pat from the wreckage. Intense, like a made-for-TV movie. But this was not TV.

At a nearby café, Pat's wife, Karen, had been eating breakfast with a friend. She'd heard the sudden loud bang of a fiery explosion and then saw the immense plume of smoke over the helipad of the hospital. Quickly and without rational thought, her mind put two and two together. She stood up and went to her car.

Pat was retrieved from the burnt and mangled fuselage and brought into the ER. The same department he had walked through minutes before.

I can only imagine the horror, confusion, and disbelief of the ER staff when the three crewmembers were wheeled into the emergency department. Emergency departments are prepared to take care of traumas. That is pretty standard. However, no one is prepared to take care of their own helicopter that crashes in their parking lot.

It was clear that all three crewmembers were significantly hurt. Each one required a team of care providers to stabilize their condition.

Dave, the flight paramedic, was severely burned and needed immediate stabilization. The heat had not only destroyed his skin but also damaged his airway. ABCs. Airway, Breathing, Circulation. Airway and breathing were a problem. To prevent his airway from closing and causing asphyxiation, the ER team quickly set up to intubate him with a breathing tube. As they prepared to put him under for the procedure, he mumbled some words.

"Tell my wife I love her."

This information is true. This isn't for drama's sake.

Pat was also in critical condition. He had been pulled from the burnt fuselage and sustained not only traumatic injuries from the impact but significant full-body burns as well. He was barely alive.

Pat's wife arrived at the ER to find her husband surrounded by staff trying to stabilize him. He was dying.

The sun was shining fully on Lake Dillon and the amphitheater. It sparkled and burned down like its job was to give my wife a tan and me a sunburn. I hadn't thought of sunscreen because I was going to a funeral.

At the time of the ceremony, Dave was still under anesthesia. Hopefully unaware of his circumstances. He would be sedated and unresponsive for the next five months.

The flight nurse was alive but in severe pain. He had broken his back and pelvis. He had neuro deficits from the injury. He, also, was unable to attend the funeral.

Father Glenn, who was presiding over the service, said that Mahany's wife had been there at the end.

"Drawn from the wreckage of the helicopter, he lay long enough there to be loved on by his wife."

He continued, "And God made sure in the last moments of his life that Karen and his friends could be there to care for him and to care for others. He did die doing what he loved, and with the ones he loved."

I became preoccupied with the view. The stage still contained the casket, family, and priests, but the lake distracted me due to its beauty. The backdrop was blatantly unaffected by the foreground. Like one had no bearing on the other. People cycled and ran by on the path behind the stage. Obviously aware of the event due to the full amphitheater, but nonetheless in their own world. It was a morning workout, nothing special.

We were well into the Mass now. I hadn't been to Mass for a while. There is something a little calming about the predictability. There is an order and a progression to the whole thing so you know what will happen next. There aren't any surprises.

My wife always asks me how I can watch a movie like *The Legend of Bagger Vance* or *Good Will Hunting* over and over. Which I do, by the way. It's because of the predictability. It gives my brain a rest.

I come home late at night from the ER and am confronted with the quiet. It's an obvious dichotomy that I'm not ready for. The quiet brings the craziness into focus, like a crisp backdrop behind a busy piece of Kandinsky artwork. It makes me uncomfortable. The quiet and the crazy, like a lake and a casket.

To escape and recover from my unsettledness, I turn on a movie. It lets me know what's coming, even if it only lasts for a couple of hours. In the movie, the struggle and emotion feel real, but, in the end, I know it will all work out. Everything will be OK. This might sound surprisingly like a four-year-old, but it is what it is. It gives my soul a rest. Kind of like church for some people.

"As we prepare to celebrate the mystery of Christ's love, let us acknowledge and ask the Lord for pardon and strength," the priest said with a customary tone.

The Catholic church is so formal.

It made me nostalgic, like a Bruce Hornsby song. As I mentioned, I went to Catholic high school, and we periodically were required to attend Mass. Back in school with my classmates, I sat in Mass completely bored. I would ponder homework, soccer practice, the girl I liked, what I was doing after school. All kinds of things, but I rarely thought about the Mass itself.

For so much of my life, I've had trouble slowing my mind. I rarely focused on the moment.

I have felt so distracted. But all that has changed.

I saw a picture of a man sitting on a bench next to his dog. They were both looking out at a beautiful view. There were thought bubbles for what each was thinking. The man had four different bubbles above his head: a car, a plane, a house, and money. The dog had only one. The dog's thought bubble was the same picture of the man and the dog sitting on the bench next to each other. Again, the image showed them enjoying the view. The caption of the photo: "Why dogs are happier than people."

"As we prepare to celebrate the mystery of Christ's love, let us acknowledge and ask the Lord for pardon and strength." What the hell does that even mean? If God expects me to talk like that, then I'm fucked.

Maybe my wife was right. Maybe it is a faith issue. Then again, maybe it isn't.

I sat contemplatively yet agitated, wishing I could have a reset. I wanted to go home and watch a movie. A movie of my choice, not some *Manchester by the Sea*, Academy Award–winning, depressing piece of crap.

Just then my wife reached over. She knows me well. Too well. She grabbed my hand and threaded her fingers into mine. I paused. She brought me into the moment. My mind stopped racing. There were no questions of *why*. I only felt the *who* in my life. She was right next to me, calming my soul. Everything I had done was so full of drive and largely self-imposed expedience. I chased so many superficial goals and truths. I needed to see loss. I needed to feel, to have my wife sit next to me and steady my soul. All that I had seen and done, my experiences of opening up and taking the red pill, had allowed me to slow down, reflect, think. It allowed me to take it in, all of it. At the moment, hand intertwined with my wife's, I felt no urgency, no rush, no goal. I stopped trying to find the good or bad. I was just knowing the moment. I took in the view—a mix of beauty and horror.

I have insomnia, and Steph has this strange calming effect on me. When I'm all worked up because it's 3:00 a.m. and I can't sleep, she lays her hand on my head. It is like she has superpowers or something. My brain slows, and the thoughts that race about are pushed back. It's like a heavy velvet cloth is thrown over the agitation. It's soothing and my mind clears. My thoughts fade to nothing. It is only a feeling of calm and gated emotion.

It brings me into my *who*.

The same thing happened at the funeral.

Her hand imparted the superpower. I softened and observed. I relaxed. I was in the moment, minus my schizophrenic mind.

THE KISS

"Sacred Stones" Samples

Dr. Sovndal," the nurse said, staring at me. "Dr. Sovndal." This time a little more forcefully.

"Yeah." I jerked my head up from the big blue ICU book.

"Do you want to do anything about the output on Mrs. Sanders? Room 325? It has dropped off a bit." She said it a bit chafed, like she didn't want or need to wait for my answer.

I stared at her for a moment. The way I stare at my wife when I've zoned out and completely missed what she said. The question hung in the air. And I continued to stare.

"I was going to give another sixty of Lasix," she said, breaking the silence.

"I should look and see if we can—"

"I think we should give the Lasix," she said firmly, like the patient, in fact, needed sixty of Lasix.

"Ah, OK, sounds good," I said, smiling. "Let's go ahead and do that. Sixty of Lasix."

"Thanks." She was gone.

The ICU is an intense place. This is where the sickest patients in the hospital get care. I felt like I had no business being there. My only option was to learn. This was sink or swim. And by *sink*, I mean getting someone killed.

Emergency medicine is a mix of all the critical elements of the different specialties. Other types of doctors say that they don't like it because ER docs aren't experts in anything. For example, ear, nose, and throat (ENT) doctors spend their entire residency focusing on the ear, nose, and throat. They are clearly experts in that specific area. Same can be said for neurologists, gynecologists, cardiologists, and any other specialists.

Emergency medicine is unique. Because in the ER, on any given day, at any time, any problem can present. Heart attack (the domain of the cardiologist), peritonsillar abscess (ENT), gunshot (trauma surgeon), baby delivery (obstetrician), dog bite to the face (plastic surgeon), overdose (toxicologist), renal failure (nephrologist), stroke (neurologist)—the list goes on and on. Because of that uncertainty, ER doctors must know how to handle anything that comes through the door. So sure, I'm no ENT, but in the middle of the night with a bleeding pharyngeal obstruction, I'm the only option the patient's got.

And that is my area of expertise. Emergency physicians are experts at initial resuscitation and stabilization of, well, everything. Our residency, which allows us to have such a wide berth, forces us to become bastard children of every other specialty. We rotate through all the various services, trying to learn as many of the critical components as possible during our short adoptive stay. I might be a trauma surgeon for five months, then I become an OB doctor, then an internist. It's difficult because you're always trying to be someone you're not. But on the flip side, it is fantastic for someone who likes stress, is easily bored, and has ADHD.

During residency, emergency medicine house staff spends considerable time in the ICU. It is a no-joke rotation. As I said, the patients are way complex and supersick. I was fortunate (sarcasm) enough to pull the straw of ICU as my first rotation during training.

I crowded in for Day One of rounds, nerves on high alert. The attending was no-nonsense, and we started briskly evaluating each patient, room by room. The amount of information was overwhelming, and I felt perpetually five steps behind. I had *MD* behind my name, but I felt out of place and in over my head.

This was serious medicine, multiple complex physiologic problems, one intertwined with the other. No textbook gave simple and straightforward answers to these patients because there weren't any. I was still trying to figure out how to write a proper SOAP progress note, not to mention figure out actual diagnoses and treatment plans.

The first day blew by like a fierce thunderstorm on the front range. I had barely caught my breath when all the team leaders started handing me their pagers. My scrub pants nearly fell down as I hooked the fifth pager onto the drawstring. Unbeknownst to me, I was on call the first night. My resident assured me I'd be fine. There was a "night float" resident "floating" around the hospital; they'd give me backup if I got into trouble. *If I got into trouble?* I was already in trouble.

Alone, in the middle of a bank of blinking and beeping monitors, I sat quietly at the doctor's desk. *Breathe in and breathe out,* I told myself. My mind was racing uncontrollably. I worked to calm down, grabbing my bouncing leg, like my arm could control it better than my brain.

Knowledge is protection. Knowledge is king. If I knew stuff, the medicine, maybe I wouldn't hurt anybody. Maybe I wouldn't be reamed on rounds by the attending the next morning. If I were smart, everyone would leave me alone. And hopefully everyone would leave alive. I decided to approach it one breath and leg bounce at a time. I opened up the blue ICU book.

The nurses in the ICU must get tired of interns. That is why my nurse was curt about the Lasix. She actually didn't need me. I would only get in the way of her taking care of the patient. She was the real doctor. I was a neophyte with a crisp white coat and a can-do attitude and not much else.

I had been reading the textbook for about a half hour when the nurse interrupted me. I had literally started on page one and hadn't made it all that far. After our brief interaction, I looked back down at the ridiculously thick book. Only a couple thousand pages to go. I knew so little. A wave of nausea came over me.

My leg started to bounce more intently.

Trying to distract myself to relieve the anxiety, I rolled my chair over and picked up one of the twenty pinkish patient binders from the chart rack. *Breathe in, breathe out.* Forget about the book's page count; the chart was a monumental amount of paperwork.

I like the author Anne Lamott. She has a book called *Bird by Bird.* In the book, her son becomes overwhelmed with a report on birds for school. She gives him sound advice. When trying to figure out everything he has to include in the paper, she says, "Bird by bird, buddy. Just take it bird by bird." I'd use her approach. Bird by bird.

Medical charts are a pain in the ass. Especially back then, because doctors' handwriting sucks. That's not a stereotype. Well, maybe it's a stereotype, but it's a true stereotype. It's hard to make anything out.

My handwriting is an exception. No really. OK, kinda. It's not "good," but at the same time it's not bad. When you first look at it you might think it is going to be a disaster to decipher. But nurses tell me, once you get through the stylistic aspect of it, it's fine. Just like reading a weird font. Most of the chart was more like trying to read the scribble of a three-year-old, on drugs.

Halfway through the binder, about forty minutes later, I decided to take another break. I set the chart down and looked up from the desk. A woman had just walked into 313. I slid my chair to the right so I could look into the room and see the patient through the glass wall. He was a young guy, thirty-eight. He wore a mask and slept restlessly, the head of his bed up at 30 degrees. Holding his hand, his wife sat in the chair at his bedside, her head resting on the rail. She was pretty. She also wore a mask. They looked like a couple that didn't belong here. They should have been at an uptown bar or hosting a dinner party at their Chelsea flat.

The patient's name was Steve. He was an up-and-coming banker who had been married to Joss for about six months. He had no medical problems save one: lung cancer. He had complained of a persistent cough and fatigue for some time but had attributed it to the stress of getting married, work, and allergies. Unfortunately, Steve's diagnosis was wrong. His doctor, on the other hand, made the correct clinical call. Bronchogenic carcinoma is a bad thing. And Steve had an aggressive form.

Looking through the window of the room, my hand resting on the thick pink chart, that was the beginning.

Day after day, I showed up to the Unit ready for work. The exhaustion was washed away by the amount of learning. I read my ass off. I asked questions. Watched procedures, then practiced them. *See one, do one, teach one.* I spoke with specialists and radiologists. I made a fool of myself countless times. I followed my attending and senior residents around like a loyal puppy. Super embarrassing when you are so close at their heels that you follow them into the bathroom. Did it. Multiple times. All those pagers? At least three of them found their way into the toilet. When you pull the string on scrub pants with seven pagers attached to them, gravity takes over.

I would come to know an unbelievable amount about bronchogenic carcinoma. I also came to learn about Steve, the person. I knew him inside and out—in many respects, literally. I learned about his entire family that held vigil at the hospital, especially his wife, Joss. Steve had grown up in upstate NY; met Joss at NYU. I knew their love story, their wedding venue, and their plans to one day move to Connecticut and start a family. Just as the medical knowledge came little by little, so did the personal knowledge about Steve and Joss.

My time in the ICU flew by. Days turned into weeks. When I first met Steve, he was full of fight. It was him against cancer, and he wasn't going to lose. He wanted it all. He wanted the knowledge, treatments, even the suffering; he wanted the "deepest darkest dogfight," just like Marcus Luttrell, the Navy SEAL of *Lone Survivor* fame.

SEALs like a good fight. So did Steve. Steve was ready to go into that shadowy place that only people fighting for their lives know about. No way did he intend on losing this battle because losing meant dying. It meant leaving Joss.

His drive and determination were "signed out" to me. The intern before me noted it and commented on it. Signing out to an oncoming intern in the ICU is an involved process. The intern leaving the service hands over all their patients to the new intern. All details and plans are spelled out so there is a consistent and continued level of care. Aside from all the medical interventions and treatments, diagnostic tests and treatment plans, one thing was abundantly clear to everyone who provided care in the ICU: Steve was a fighter.

Steve and Joss monitored everything, every day. I would do rounds with the medical team, and then I'd do personal rounds with Steve and Joss.

Because of Steve's weakened state and the chemotherapy, no one entered his room without a mask, lest they pass on some potentially life-threatening germs. It was odd to see his family, especially Joss, without their masks in the hallway. I had grown so accustomed to their covered faces that they didn't seem themselves without a hidden nose and mouth.

From the moment I assumed his care, his progress, or lack thereof, was evident. Sitting at the central desk, reading chart 313 on my first day, I didn't know much. But I knew this: the notes, labs, and images looked bad. With each passing week, highlighted by each passing day, he grew more and more tired. He became thin and wasted. He tried to eat but couldn't keep the weight on. I wrote orders for supplementation, but the effort was in vain. His numbers worsened. Some went up and others down, but none seemed to be going in the right direction. He looked like an athlete who had just finished a marathon, all the time.

Steve was losing ground.

It was a Sunday. The reason I know that is because the hospital was quiet, without the normal daily traffic. I also remember being frustrated that I had to be there. I had come into work the day before and had been on call. I would be leaving after rounds this morning, but that was still hours away. I woke from an early morning nap and went to the cafeteria to get some coffee. The fact that there were only a few people there invigorated me. It meant I was going home . . . soon. I could pretend to be a normal person in New York, if only for an afternoon. I hadn't seen my wife in three days. When I had gotten off work the day before I started call, she had been out with work friends, and I was so exhausted I had just gone to bed. Maybe later today we could take a walk in Riverside Park and take in the view of the Hudson.

I read through my notes as I sipped my coffee. Rounds would happen in an hour. After taking a few minutes to organize my thoughts, I headed back to the Unit to review the test results and finish rounding on my patients.

Joss was in Steve's room, as usual.

"How's it going?" I said it with a positive tone.

"OK," he said.

He never said, "OK." He always gave some sort of positive answer, like "Great," or "Better than yesterday." The Disney way.

His initial exam seemed consistent. He was wasted away, thin, with pale, scaly skin. The port on his chest looked good. "Clean, dry, and intact," as my note said. However, when I got to his lungs, they seemed a bit coarser. There were decreased breath sounds at both bases with significant rales. That snorkel with water in it that I mentioned earlier. There was more fluid in his lungs.

Steve had had routine labs drawn that morning, as well as a CT. There was no report by the radiologist so I called him on the phone. Things were worse. Fluid had built up in Steve's lungs and become loculated. His labs were also off.

I waited for my turn on rounds. Room 310, 311, and then 312. We pulled up short, in the hallway gap between rooms.

There was a small crowd gathered, which was typical. Attending, the nurse for that patient, three interns from the service, one of whom was me, a couple of junior residents, a senior resident, a nutritionist, and a social worker. All of us formed a semicircle as each intern gave their report to the team.

My presentation started with a brief summary and our current game plan. I recapped the CT and labs that I had mulled over earlier. The attending and senior confirmed what I had already figured out, even as a first year. The data was worse than expected. In fact, the information was downright dismal. The cancer had become more aggressive and had spread, despite our best efforts. Despite Steve's efforts. In addition to the messed-up findings in his lungs, it was now in his bones and liver. All his systems were failing. Cancer is like Napoleon on the march, relentless. It knows exactly where to hit its enemy.

As an intern, you manage patients primarily, which means you are their first-line provider. Your senior resident and the attending give oversight, but they are managing a larger volume of patients. It is a pyramid-type structure. Attending oversees everyone, then senior resident, then junior resident, and finally intern. Due to the structure, the intern spends the most one-on-one time at the bedside. It's the intern who is in the trenches, who really gets to know the patient and family. In part, because the intern has the time, but also because the intern doesn't know enough to get out of the way.

The attending told me he wanted a "care meeting" with the patient and his family. In Steve's situation, it was going to be an end-of-life discussion. Hospice, comfort measures, treatment at home, things of that nature. No more plans to search and destroy. This was a surrender. Napoleon had won. The plan was to make Steve comfortable. That's all my esteemed and learned attending had to offer. That's all my Columbia education and perfect MCAT score had to offer.

We started to move, the circle uncoiled, and the train of doctors began walking to the next room, 314. I interrupted the flow briefly to ask my attending a question.

"What do I tell them?"

He looked at me as if I had grown an additional arm.

"What do you mean, 'What do I tell them?'" He paused, looking at me over the top of his glasses.

I just stared, like when I gave the Lasix, like when I piss off my wife.

"You go in there and tell them there is a care meeting in an hour and a half."

"But they'll want to know the results. I mean, when I go in the room, they'll want to know the results then," I said, searching for an excuse that meant I wasn't going to be the one. That this wasn't going to be on me.

"Just give them the results. You're their doctor, right?" Still looking at me with his chin down and eyebrows up, like I was a moron and he was an asshole. He pushed his glasses up and moved on. Everyone followed, but I lagged, looking through the window, watching Joss tending to Steve.

We finished rounds, and the other intern asked if I was taking off to go home.

"No, I have the care meeting." I didn't care about going home anymore. My spirit was broken. Like a depressed patient with anhedonia, I wasn't sure what I would do even if I did leave this wretched place.

I entered their room, mask on as always.

"What did it show?" Steve said. His voice was clearly tired.

I had read somewhere to just give the bad news. Don't beat around the bush. A bullet to the head is better than five to the chest and bleeding to death.

I pulled up a chair and sat. "Not good." I paused and gave a sympathetic smile, which they obviously didn't see.

"It spread. It looks like it's all over. The PET scan lit up in your back, your spine, your kidneys, and liver. It also looks—"

"I got it," Steve said, interrupting me. He was calm. He already knew the results. Deep down, he knew.

I had expected a defiant response, a Steve response. But I didn't get one.

"I got it." That was all he said, again. I leaned forward onto my elbows and lowered my head.

"Steve, I think we just need to regroup," Joss started. "We have a care meeting in an hour. We can see if . . ." Steve interrupted again, calmly, quietly.

"Hey man, can you give us a minute?" he said. I looked up.

His face, around his eyes and forehead, had lost tension. His eyes had a sad surrender. A look of relief.

"Yes. Absolutely. Sure." I mistimed my response so it sounded awkward and overeager. Then I hesitated, awkwardly, again. I stood up and stopped at the door. I fumbled my delivery. "Sorry.... Sorry, I wanted different news."

"Yeah"—a slight laugh—"me too." Steve was fixated on Joss.

I left the room and sat down at the same center desk where I had first peered into his room. I took off my white coat. That thing was so goddamn hot and constricting.

Fuck that coat.

I leaned back, took a deep breath, and slowly spun around in the chair. As it completed its revolution, I looked into their room. I could see them talking, Joss more animated than Steve. I felt like I was invading their space but couldn't help it. Like driving by a car accident. Or at the funeral.

He gently grabbed Joss's hand, and she seemed to quiet. He must have the magical touch too. She sat down again. His other hand came up and pulled off his mask, dropping it on the floor.

He leaned his head back on his pillow. With his eyes welling up, he smiled at his wife. I hadn't seen that smile. Ever. Then he chuckled, like she had said something funny. With deliberate motion, he touched her again, pushing the hair back over her ear. He slipped off the elastic band holding her mask.

It looked like the ICU air smelled fantastic, like the beach at Bodega Bay.

Tears rolled down Joss's cheeks.

I felt a rage building inside me. Like an anxiety attack forged with the wrath of a caged animal.

It was fear. It was death. It was room 313. It was fucking God.

I wanted to scream.

But as I continued to look, my rage started to calm.

Room 313 was the antidote.

It was the cause *and* the cure.

Breathe in, breathe out. Big forward, small back.

Steve and Joss were talking. They were calm. They seemed at peace.

In that moment, they seemed happy. Sad but happy at the same time, and I don't know if that makes any sense at all.

They kissed. It was passionate, without the hustle. And yes, I was watching. Long, slow, and consuming. The kind of kiss a princess would dream about.

Joss stood up and moved onto his bed. She lay down inside his grip and scooted close. He caved around her.

I left the ICU and got another cup of coffee, this one from the trailer outside.

When I came back they were still lying there. They didn't move for a really long time.

The care meeting went as planned, with a mask-less Steve and Joss.

"I want to go home." It was put simply and then acknowledged by my attending.

I wrote the discharge order, "DC home."

Joss packed up their suitcases and belongings.

It's a cliché to leave the hospital in a wheelchair. Unless, of course, you need a wheelchair.

"Let me help you guys down," I said, grabbing the suitcase. I followed behind as she pushed.

We made it to the front entrance, and she left to get the car. I stood there not knowing what to say. I was standing with a dead man.

"Yankees might pull it off this year," he said.

"Probably," I said. Joe Torre, Alex Rodriguez, Derek Jeter. They probably would. I hate the Yankees.

We got him in the car, and Joss walked around to the other side.

She gave a quick, distracted wave like she didn't mean it and slid in through the driver's door. I saw a subtle sigh as she grabbed the steering wheel. There was no monumental goodbye. No closure to the weeks we had spent together. Merely a door shutting and a car driving away.

"Bye," I said to myself, my hand frozen in the air.

I never saw them again.

RED BULL

"Summer, Highland Falls" Billy Joel

The first time I drank Red Bull was at a Bonefish concert in Aspen. A couple of buddies and I had flown there from California during residency. Arriving at the concert, on no sleep, with only beef jerky, Coca-Cola, and Red Vines in our system (convenience store road trip stop), we started to drink Red Bull vodkas like they were going out of style. "One foot on the gas, one on the brake," my friend Tim said as he handed me the drink combo. Next thing I knew I was in the middle of a mosh pit with a bunch of dudes much bigger and crazier than me. The accelerator won. The next morning was not pretty. So much for a killer ski day.

Since then I've learned a more appropriate dosing and timing of Red Bull. Too soon and you flame out, too late and you can't sleep. And too much, you end up in a mosh pit. I had finished all my training and moved to Colorado. At this point my wife and I had two awesome boys and a sweet house up one of the canyons in Boulder. I was working as a full-fledged ER doc in our city's only hospital. Just what I had planned. Tonight, I was just about ready to crack open an eight-ouncer since the ER was pretty much under control.

"Shannon, I can't believe you don't think the Rock is hot," the nurse said, smiling. She thought he was the most attractive man ever. Kelly supported her initial statement, "He's a professional athlete! He's ripped, an actor, and a totally nice guy."

"Really? Nice?" I scrunched up my face. "Didn't know you knew him."

"No, I just know he is. He's so sweet in his interviews," she concluded.

"Oh, well. That makes sense then." I laughed.

The ER had slowed, so we had a small crowd of staff joining the debate. I looked at the group of female nurses, knowing this would get them going, and said matter-of-factly, "I'm a way better catch than the Rock." There was an uproar of laughter.

"Really?" Kelly smiled.

"Absolutely," I confidently responded, standing and strutting just a little.

Before Kelly and the other nurses could rip into me, the bay doors opened. An EMS crew rolled through in a rush. They had a little old lady in significant respiratory distress. Conversation over, we were back in business.

"No call?" the charge nurse asked.

"Sorry." The paramedic fumbled with his wires as he prepared to move the patient to our bed. "The radio isn't working. We didn't have a chance. We were at Manor Crest, right down the street."

"What's her deal?" I asked.

"They found her laying on the floor in the dining room." The paramedic cleared his throat after he said it.

By the time they moved her onto our bed, she was limp and blue. I moved to the head of the bed and looked at her face, now upside down in perspective.

"Can you bag her?"

"It's not working," said the medic.

"Did you look?" I asked.

"Yeah, something nasty is in there, but I couldn't get it."

The nurse attempted to ventilate the woman as I clicked a laryngoscope blade to extension. The patient was so limp this would be a "crash" intubation. We use different treatment pathways, like "crash," "failed," and "difficult" airway, to handle patients with breathing issues. Ideally, we induce, paralyze, and sedate patients in a process called RSI (rapid sequence intubation). This patient was so close to checking out I didn't think we had time to draw up and give the drugs.

Her O2 saturation was in the 50s. A low-pitch chirp played out on the monitor. The lower the pitch, the lower the oxygen saturation.

I popped out her false teeth and slid in the laryngoscope blade. As I looked I saw a big "something" blocking my view. I focused. I couldn't quite make out what it was. I felt the warmth of adrenaline surge through my body. It felt familiar.

I repositioned the laryngoscope, and my brain began to process what I was seeing. Time was critical.

If the oxygen saturation drops, you can survive to a point. Oxygen saturation refers to the amount of oxygen molecules bound to the hemoglobin molecule. The majority of oxygen in your body is transported in this bound form. The rest (to a lesser extent) is free floating in the bloodstream. We use oxygen saturation as a quick indicator of how much oxygen your blood is delivering to the tissue.

If the saturation gets lower than 80 percent, the dissociation curve of delivering oxygen to the tissue drops like it jumped off a cliff. Cells start to suffocate, which means the patient suffocates. A saturation in the 50s was dodgy, real dodgy. And the number was dropping.

"Hand me the forceps," I demanded softly, without raising my voice.

Caroline briskly slid open the third drawer of the resuscitation tool chest and handed me some Magill's.

The beep of the saturation monitor got deeper in tone, meaning the saturation was dropping.

I worked the handle of the laryngoscope, coordinating with the Magill's. I couldn't get the rounded end of the forceps to find purchase on the foreign body. *Man, this is slippery.*

"Come on, one time," I said softly under my breath. No luck. "Get out the cric kit, please."

I figured that might start to freak everyone out so I said it softly, and with a *please*. Cutting into someone's neck, placing a breathing tube through the cricoid cartilage, didn't occur often. I wasn't convinced I'd have to do it, but since my patient was already on borrowed time I wanted the ball rolling. One more shot at grabbing this thing, and then I was all over this lady's neck like white on rice.

I set down the Magill's and grabbed the bougie. It's a long, blue, flexible, and pliable tubelike device. I added a little extra bend to the end, hoping to make a hook. Since it has such a small diameter, I was able to slip by the edge of the obstruction, using the release of surrounding soft tissue. Once the bougie's tip passed the obstruction distally, I gave a twist, hoping to engage the hook. I pulled back with a quick movement. It didn't totally dislodge the foreign body, but popped it up enough so the Magill's could find purchase. I quickly discarded the bougie and grabbed the forceps. I twisted my forearm and wrist. This time the Magill's slipped around the whitish-green clump that was damming up her trachea.

"Here it is," Carolyn said, plopping down the cric kit on the Mayo stand at the bedside. I ignored her.

A gentle grip was the best grip. I learned this from my buddy Allen. He taught me this with chopsticks. "The trick," he had said, "is not muscling the end of the sticks together. You have to be gentle and just barely put pressure on the piece of sushi." I used the same technique with my forceps. Not too much pressure, not too little. Just right.

"Got it," I exclaimed softly and matter-of-factly. I pulled out a big chunk of food pinched in the end of my forceps. It was a piece of soft, partially chewed chicken that looked like it was covered in a pesto sauce. But that's just a guess.

As I held the instrument up, the woman took a gasping breath. She started to breathe as the nurse replaced the bag valve mask. Her color began to return, and the chirp of the O2 sat monitor reassuringly elevated its pitch.

I continued to manage her airway, but she seemed to be improving. After a minute or two, Kelly came over to the Mayo stand to pick up the cric kit. I leaned over, smiling smugly, and said softly, "Let's see the Rock do that!"

She didn't seem to be overly amused.

No sooner had I removed my gloves and washed my hands than the tech stuck her head in the room and told me my wife was on the line.

"OK, tell her I'll call her back in a few. Thanks." I had just listened to my patient's lungs, and they sounded clear. The saturation monitor was scribing away at 98 percent. She was going to be fine for now. She started to wake up. Just like that. Maybe an aspiration pneumonia was in her future, but for now, she was improving and opened her eyes.

"We're going to watch you for a little bit. Make sure you're OK." I said it like I was talking to a deaf person. I wasn't totally sure if she could hear me or not. I put my hand on her shoulder and gave a smile like she didn't almost die. I wrote down a couple of orders and asked for a chest X-ray.

I walked back to the doc box and sat down in front of my computer and phone. My mood changed.

I had been married to Jane for nearly ten years, but for the past year, things had not been good. I remember meeting her in Shakespeare class. She sat down next to me, and naturally, I struck up a conversation. We did the standard introductions and small talk. Then the conversation took a turn I hadn't expected.

"I haven't been feeling so well," Jane said.

"Really? That sucks," I said as compassionately as possible.

"I think I have worms." It came out no-nonsense, like, obviously, that was the source of her problem.

"Worms?" I couldn't help but smile.

She realized how it sounded and smiled as well. "I just got back from Africa, and I think I got some parasite or something."

That was it. *I think I have worms.*

We stayed married during all my medical training, and that is saying something. Medical school followed by internship followed by residency. I'm sure that being married to someone in medical training is no cakewalk. But I thought we were beating the odds. Doctors have a ridiculous divorce rate, and so far so good, I had thought.

I went into the doctor's cubicle to make the call. I picked up the receiver and punched the numbers. "Hi." I tried to sound as upbeat as possible.

"Hi. Can we talk when you get home?" She didn't sound pissed. That was a plus. No small talk, just the question.

"Is everything OK?" I asked.

"Yes. I think it's going to be fine. Everything will be fine."

My Spidey-Sense was going off. The way she said it was creepy, but maybe I was just reading into it. I had the impression she was saying she'd be fine if we *didn't* work it out. It felt odd. My Spidey-Sense had been wrong before . . . but rarely.

"Will you pick up some cigarettes on the way home?" she asked, as if the request was normal.

"Ah"—I paused for only a moment—"sure." I didn't want to add to what already seemed like an edgy conversation.

My wife was all about cool. The first time she showed up at my door in college, my roommate Jon didn't know what to make of her. She wore all black, work boots, and a mechanic jacket with a patch ("Stan") sewn on the front. When I came to the door, Jon turned and walked toward me making a funny face and mouthing *Who's that?* She wasn't my normal type. She looked tougher, edgier, and like more trouble than my past girlfriends. When we started dating she had smoked, but then quickly gave it up because she knew I had no interest in kissing an ashtray.

Cigarettes. Hmmm.

My shift ended at eleven. I finished up my last patient, stopped off at the gas station, and arrived home about a quarter past midnight. She had waited up for me only once before, my first shift in residency, when we lived in Palo Alto. After that I had become accustomed to coming home to a quiet and sleepy house. She met me in the kitchen, grabbed two beers, and said, "Let's go on the deck."

It was a beautiful night. We lived in an awesome house with a deck that extended out as the roof of the garage. The Colorado foothills were impressive.

Halloween-style clouds whisked across the full moon. They were ominous. I could see the silhouette of the mountains and trees scattered in the distance.

My wife lit up a cigarette as I uncomfortably took a sip of my beer.

Damn, that view was amazing.

"I don't love you." She took a slow drag and said it so nonchalantly that I was caught off guard. Her look was calm, which made it even more cruel.

The moment had come slow but fast. Big forward, small back.

"I never loved you," she said dryly. The same way you'd say, "My family comes from Germany."

PARIS

"Chances" Five for Fighting

Paris is amazing. I stood and looked at Stephanie on the Pont des Arts. We'd be lucky if the bridge didn't collapse due to all the padlocks. I was five years out from my divorce. As I stood over the Seine, I felt something different. I was vulnerable yet strong at the same time. I was excited yet grounded. I felt this woman was strange, different, in a good way. Like nothing I had experienced before.

I'm sure some of you may feel like I jumped ahead. By now, you have to know that the ADHD takes over sometimes. Who is this guy who is now talking about a bridge in Paris with a girl named Steph? Perhaps you want to know all the gritty details of the last five years. I get it. It seems reasonable. You want to know if I almost lost it and started using crack? Did I drink too much? Did I quit medicine? All reasonable questions.

I had a writer friend, Will, read this book while I was working on it. I know that is what he was thinking. Here are the comments that he sent me on this section. He was hoping for more, so he decided to do a little writing for me.

> "Love had not worked for me. I was a single father, was angry, afraid of dating, took heroin to cope, embezzled money. Then an angel appeared, when I crashed my Ferrari. I woke up in the hospital and Steph was by my bedside in her sexy cargo pants stained with my blood. Her eyelashes were singed from when she pulled me from the burning wreckage."
>
> Something like that.
>
> —Will

So let's get this out of the way. *No* on the crack. *Yes* on the drinking, but nothing crazy. I didn't become an alcoholic or anything. And, regarding medicine, almost, but no.

Getting divorced sucks. I mean it s-u-c-k-s! I was damaged, for a long time. I feel really sorry for the first few women I dated after that. (You know who you are. . . . I'm sorry.) It couldn't have been good.

The nature of betrayal meant there were a lot of emotions—almost all of them bad. Bitterness, anger, finger-pointing, confusion. Just like someone dying, these emotions are like a black hole. I found myself circling closer and closer to oblivion for more than two years.

Talk about having your heart ripped out from your chest. *I never loved you.* It cost me a lot, not just in pain, loneliness, and suffering, but in money for therapy. I can only make light of it because it happened so long ago, close to thirteen years now.

But at the time, there was nothing light about it. It was all-encompassing. Devastating. I had planned to become an ER doc and move to Colorado. All the pieces had fallen into place, except one. The most important one: family.

So many things could have been done differently on my end. The sheer volume of work in medical school and residency consumed me. I was just unavailable. Maybe that caused her to look elsewhere. I could barely hold myself together during all the emotions of people living and dying right in front of me. There was a long while where I lost a little of myself just trying to survive.

But this monumental failure has ultimately saved me. Like dropping out of the Academy, I never could have suspected where it would lead me. I needed to shrink down and shrivel up to ultimately grow and broaden my horizons. I needed to become worse to be better. Specifically, I needed to become a better man. Otherwise I would be nowhere good enough for my kids or my wife, Stephanie.

Not a day goes by, even this far out, that I'm not aware that I have been divorced. It's impossible to forget when you are co-parenting kids.

But the view changes with time. Our two sons are phenomenal, and if I had to do it all over again to get them, I would in a heartbeat. Experience opens up emotion and capacity, and today I am nowhere near the man I was then.

I had a lot of focused time with my kids. The space allowed me to figure out how to be a complete dad, meaning, they were totally mine during my 50-50 time, and it forced me to grow. I could completely focus on our new family, and it was impressively enlightening.

So, I wish I had a cool story of crashing a Ferrari and being pulled out of the flames by a beautiful blond. That would make a better book. Maybe in a different life, but more on that later.

Since I don't have any really cool stories, let's stick with the overwhelming fact that the woman I loved didn't love me back. It took me a long time to recover.

But that's what makes this bridge so good.

The Pont des Arts sits southeast of the Musée d'Orsay on Quai Voltaire. It connects the St. Germain district to the Louvre. From the bridge looking east, you can see the Seine split into two branches that flow around the Île de la Cité. It's cool because that's where the Cathédrale Notre-Dame de Paris sits.

I want you to know. I don't speak French. I just Googled the hell out of it.

The sun had already set, and the lights of the city were reflecting off the river. Steph leaned over the railing to watch the water slowly roll underneath. I could see the top of Notre Dame peeking over the other buildings, but my attention was drawn to Stephanie. She is indeed beautiful.

The "love lock" bridge is covered with thousands of padlocks. Steph had arrived in Paris earlier that day, and after eating dinner, we ended up on this bridge. Steph was enthralled with all the locks. I conjured a story about couples getting married in Paris and then padlocking their "love" to the bridge. Just then, a couple came riding over on bikes. The woman was in a wedding dress and the man in an all-black suit. They stopped their bikes and attached their lock.

"See," was all I had to say. I didn't really know that it was a "thing," but I can put two and two together.

Steph was smiling ear to ear. I barely could call her my girlfriend, but here we were in Paris standing on the padlock bridge.

As a doctor, I worked for a professional cycling team. I know I'm jumping around. I apologize again, but I can't find my Ritalin. (Just kidding). I promise it will all come back together—divorce, Steph, a bridge in France, and cycling. Just bear with me.

Remember earlier when I talked about getting into cycling when I was an undergrad at UC Davis? During my time there I had become obsessed with racing. It helped me cope with quitting and my anxiety about the quality of person I was.

I think my internal fire and vexation burned hot. I had a fair amount of success racing. So much so that I took time off from school just to focus on training and racing. I wanted to beat the likes of Greg LeMond and Miguel Indurain. Lance wasn't really a "thing" yet.

My time racing paid off, but not the way I thought. I never got to take down the greats in a competition or climb on the podium at the Tour de France. I just wasn't that fast. But I did get the next-best thing, at least in my opinion. I became a team doctor for a professional cycling team. The same way I didn't become a fighter pilot. Rather, I got to be a doctor on a medical helicopter.

This was due, in part, to my divorce. Because I only had the kids half-time, I found a freedom. And I was ready for something new. I wanted an escape. Due to people I had met racing, I was given the opportunity to help with a domestic cycling team as their doctor. Lo and behold, that team blew up in a big way. It became a UCI Pro Tour Cycling team run by Jonathan Vaughters, previous teammate of Lance Armstrong. It became known as the "clean" team.

Here is the premise of pro cycling as a business. These famous professional athletes ride their bikes all over the world as moving billboards. The team sells signage. Essentially advertising space. I worked for Slipstream Sports. That's the company that actually ran the team. However, the public knew us as TIAA-CREF, Team Garmin, Team Cannondale, and EF Education First Pro Cycling Team, to name a few. The name changes because of sponsorship, but the supporting corporation, Slipstream, remains the scaffolding that actually holds everything together.

Back to the "clean" team. As many of you already know, cycling is not known as the cleanest sport. I would argue that wherever there is money there is doping. MLB and the NFL are worth a lot more than the UCI. The reason that you hear so much more about cycling than about the NFL, is that cycling is trying hard to clean up the sport, and they are willing to suffer the consequences. Hence, the bad press after positive doping tests. But that is a topic for a different book.

(As an aside, I had considered writing a book called *Doping for Idiots*, yellow cover and all, but decided against it. I thought it wouldn't help my career as a cycling doctor. I decided to write a couple of training books instead.)

As a business, Slipstream was built on the premise of selling advertising space with the "good guys." The ones who didn't dope. In our team meetings, the discussions weren't *win at all costs*. The discussion was *stay clean at all costs*. It was a novel way to do business. The athletes weren't pushed to dope so they could win. They were pushed to be clean and compete so we could sell ad space.

I want to clarify: I never doped anyone. No way. With Slipstream I was never asked or pressured to do it. That's why I loved working with the team. But the reason I could write my idiot book was that I am not an idiot. Any professional team doctor could tell you how an athlete is doping and getting away with it—because they are a doctor and they understand the rules of the sport. I just wanted to make clear to everyone reading this that doping wasn't my thing.

Cycling is a European sport. Sure, we have it in the US, but in Europe, it is big. Like the NFL, MLB, and the NBA. I always thought that being a US pro cyclist would be just the right amount of fame. You could be a big-time sports celebrity whenever you were racing overseas. But you could come home, be back in the US, and be nearly anonymous. No one would bother you, except for the rare cycling fan, which might be good if you were on a date or something or trying to impress your kids.

The best comparison I have to being a star athlete occurred on Pearl Street, in Boulder. I was on a date—during that five-year period between my divorce and Steph—and we were strolling on the pedestrian mall after dinner. The conversation was going pretty well when we were interrupted by a homeless guy. He was lying next to the water feature and the flower bed.

He looked up from his reclined position and said, "Hey, I know you!"

Always good on a date to be recognized by a homeless dude.

"You saved my life." He started to sit up. "No, really, you saved my life. High five."

I smiled and tried to scoot out of the way so I wouldn't have to actually high-five him.

"Thanks, man."

We kept walking, and my date asked if that was true.

"Yeah, it's true."

It was like I had paid him or something.

OK, here is where I start to tie it all back together. Thanks for bearing with me. I had known Stephanie for a few years, but it was only professional. Not like that. Get your mind out of the gutter. She was a firefighter-paramedic in the city where I was an ER doctor.

We would chat when she'd drop patients off. A family friend asked us once, "Let me get this straight. You guys flirted while doing CPR or something?"

No, we never flirted while doing CPR, but the ER is no different from any other workplace. After she'd finish signing out one of her patients, she'd stop by the docs' workstation to say hello.

I remember the first time I saw her in normal clothes. My PA (physician's assistant), Noel, had gone out for her birthday with some girlfriends. She was showing me pictures of their night out.

"Who is that?!" I said looking at the picture, raising my eyebrows.

"You know her. That's Stephanie," Noel said.

I continued to stare.

"It's Stephanie," Noel said again.

"Paramedic Stephanie?" I responded.

"Yeaaahhh." Noel said it with that intonation that girls use when you're being an idiot.

I'm not saying Stephanie doesn't look good in her polyester paramedic uniform, but girls' clothes take her to a whole new level.

About a week later, after Steph dropped off a patient, she swung into the docs' cubby with her typical cheery self. I didn't let her know about the work clothes/regular clothes thing. During the conversation, I made a comment about our coffee. I don't really mind the ER coffee. It's grungy and expected. But I was making conversation with a girl, so I told her she was lucky that she was "free." She could drive around in the ambulance or fire engine, go to any coffee shop in her service area. We were stuck with the instant machine.

Twenty minutes later she had dropped a large cup of coffee at my desk. She didn't even wait to chat with me. I think Noel must have told her about the picture from the birthday and the "hot" comment. That was the beginning.

Over the next two years we went on roughly four dates, one every six months. Neither of us wanted to move too fast, for different reasons. She knew I was divorced with kids. And old. I knew she was a fiery, free-spirited firefighter-paramedic. And young. The way our birthdays matched, for about a month, she was twenty-nine while I had just turned forty. I like to tell people I was in my forties and she was in her twenties.

On a side note, her mom ended up marrying a guy who was about eleven years younger than she was. That puts Steph's father and me at about the same age. Ken's a great guy. But, yeah, a little weird.

I was getting ready to leave Boulder for work at the Tour de France with the cycling team. At the end of the race our team has a big party. I should say a huge party. It is a pro team-style gala with pomp, excess, VIPness, and all. Pharrell and N.E.R.D were going to be the private band. That kind of party.

The previous two years I had attended solo. I'm not complaining. It's pretty fun being a single guy at a Tour de France party, but this year I wanted to go with a date. I just had to figure out how to make that work.

There were some logistical issues. I didn't want the girl to necessarily think this was serious. What if she came all the way to Paris and we didn't hit it off? That would be awkward. At the same time, who would drop everything and come to Paris on such short notice? I was leaving in less than a week.

I discussed my extraordinary dating dilemma with Noel.

"You should ask Steph! She'd be perfect!" she said. "You know you'll have a blast. She's totally cool. Maybe she'll even *like* you, like you."

I'm not making this up. Noel can confirm. I kid you not, just then, Steph walked into the ER.

"Hi guys!" She strolled over to our desks. "Hi, Dr. Sovndal." She drew it out in her sassy kind of way as she leaned close to my desk.

"Hey, Steph." I paused for only a moment, Noel and I realizing the timing. "You *would* be perfect," I said.

With her classic huge smile: "Perfect"—mimicking me—"for what?"

Noel sat there, entertained by the show.

"Want to go to Paris?" I tried to play it off like this was a typical request.

Steph responded with a laugh.

"I've got to go work at the Tour." Steph looked at me like she had no idea what I was talking about.

"It's a big bike race. And the team is going to have a big . . . a huge . . . party at the end of the race. It's in Paris. Want to go?"

Steph chuckled again. She thought I was kidding. She knew nothing about cycling.

I added, "You might not remember me in ten years, but I guarantee you, you'll remember this party."

This is one of the many reasons I love Steph. Right then and there she sat at a computer terminal and started searching for flights.

A few minutes later: "Two grand!" She spun and looked at me. "You paying?"

"You get the ticket, but then I'll take care of everything else," I replied.

Before you crucify me for not paying, let me explain. I didn't want her to go to Paris just because she wanted a free trip. I wanted her to go because she was interested. I wanted to test the water. See if she actually *wanted* to go with me.

Noel chimed in, "Yeah, you should go. You could meet a professional cyclist or something. You might meet the man of your dreams."

Freakin' Noel.

Steph and I talked for a bit longer. Our chat ended when I was called over to see a patient. She took off back to work.

Less than fifteen minutes later, I got a text:
I'll go. That's what credit cards are for.

We met every day before I left to go to the race. Coffee, beer, a quick chat—it didn't really matter. It was more that I just had to see her. I had that nervous, excited feeling every time I was near her. Even hearing her voice on the phone was captivating.

She drove me to the airport. I remember she was short on fuel. "I got to get some gas." I felt worried, the way you feel worried about a new girlfriend. Just a note, she wasn't my girlfriend . . . yet. I didn't want her stranded on the way home. One, I was just plain worried about her safety, being stranded. But two, she'd be waiting on the side of the road, then some guy would stop, swoop in, and steal the girl of my dreams. If I had seen her on the side of the road, I would have stopped to help.

I'd be in France for a couple of weeks before she came over. I had never kissed her, held her hand, or anything, and on the drive, I kept thinking I should reach over and touch her, do something. But I didn't.

We pulled up to the United terminal and I climbed out, grabbing my bag. She stepped out of the car to say goodbye. Again, I thought, *Should I kiss her?* I gave her a hug.

I saw her looking out her window as I turned back while walking into the terminal. She looked beautiful, even in the polyester.

It seemed like an eternity. I was at the most exciting bike race in the world, but it dragged on like our pastor on Christmas Eve. My phone bill was going to be horrendous—this was pre WhatsApp and Viber, but man, it felt like the best money I had ever spent.

Stephanie arrived in Paris the night before the final day of the Tour. I had conned my way into leaving Bordeaux with a team car the day she arrived. The rest of the team was due to arrive in Paris the next day by train.

My best friend, Allen, working with another pro team, had already arrived in Paris, and he met her when she got in from the airport. He took her out to dinner with some other friends. To this day, she still has Allen's name in her phone as "Allen, Paris" because she didn't know who he was at the time.

I pulled into the valet of the hotel, black Skoda car with the standard Argyle shrink-wrapped logos and sponsors. I could barely contain myself. It had been torture. I couldn't wait to see her face-to-face.

I hurried down to the restaurant where Allen and the group were eating. As I walked in, I caught her looking at me from the far side of the table.

Dinner was fantastic—Paris, the end of the race, my best friend, and Steph.

I told Allen the next day, "I'm going to marry her . . . if she isn't crazy. If she's like this when we get back home, I'm going to marry her."

We finished our meal and Allen and the others said their goodbyes. Steph and I were finally alone. We started to walk down the street in Paris. I slid my hand into hers, and we just kept walking. We acted like we had been doing this for fifty years.

We walked for a long while, heading down Rue Royale and across on Quai des Tuileries. We were talking and taking in Paris. Finally, we turned at this bridge, the Pont des Arts, in front of the Louvre. Steph squatted down and looked at the locks. Some had Sharpie-written names and dates, while others were engraved. She seemed so happy. She read some of them aloud.

I had moved close as she talked, and when she stood up, we were face-to-face. It sounds totally contrived, but it's not. I had never seen anything so beautiful in my entire life. I leaned in and gave her a kiss. The kiss. Passionate, without the hustle. Maybe a *little* hustle. Right there on the bridge, in Paris.

STEPHANIE

"True Companion" Marc Cohn

The Champs-Élysées, the ultimate day of the Tour de France. Because Steph didn't know anything about cycling before she came over, she had no idea what to expect. *Just a bunch of guys in bike shorts,* she thought. The sheer scale of one of the most famous sporting events in the world totally eluded her. Maybe you're like Steph and don't know, but the Tour de France is epic. Beyond Lance Armstrong and doping. It is a sight to see.

At the finish line, and along most of the route, it is a complete zoo. There are unbelievable crowds. It's patriotic French, yet at the same time an international event. The bikes, team cars, mechanics' trucks, team buses, and press corps, combined with the security, race control, and fanatical fans, make for a menagerie of congestion, vivid colors, excessive noise, and clamorous excitement.

I had her hook up with some of the cyclists' wives and girlfriends so she'd get to the finish OK. I had to work in the team car, so I wouldn't be seeing her until the finishing laps.

The laps around the Champs-Élysées are fun for everyone—including the riders, team staff, and fans. As part of the tradition of the last day, VIPs get rides in the team cars for a lap. This year we also got hot pizza, during the race, in the car. A *soigneur* had handed it to us during one of the stops.

A giant pit stop is formed at the Place de la Concorde. The cars come flying in from the cobbles, screeching tires slamming to a halt. One VIP is pushed out, and another is shoved in. Then, gunning the throttle, the car shoots out of the pits like it's a Formula 1 race, hoping not to have lost too much ground following the peloton. The cars still needed to provide support to the riders—fix flats, give food and water, etc.—so we couldn't let ourselves get too far behind the pack. And if you haven't seen it, the riders aren't going slow. They are traveling around 40–50 kph most of the way.

I arranged to have Steph show up at the pit stop. She was going to go from not knowing anything about cycling to partaking in one of the most exclusive experiences for a cycling fan, riding in a team car, on the Champs-Élysées no less. Our Team Garmin car was booked up with sponsors. However, a buddy on SAXO had space. And I don't think he complained when he saw a blond chick hopping into the front seat of his car.

Steph was radiant when we met up after the race at the team bus. Everyone was celebrating. Champagne, crowds, laughter, relief. Everything that you'd expect after the finish.

We returned to the hotel only to be rushed out by a bus to our private party under the perfectly lit Eiffel Tower. Pharrell killed it. Better than you'd see on *The Voice*.

A couple of days later, we were lying on the grass in front of the Eiffel Tower. I had Steph's head nestled into my shoulder. The weather was warm, there were a few scattered clouds, and the Tower rose up in front of us, over our toes, like the Iron Giant.

Then we heard a laugh. A familiar laugh, from Allen. He had seen us lying there in the grass. He was also taking a few days of much-needed R&R with his girlfriend. He snapped a picture without us even knowing. He took it from grass level, aiming slightly upward along the horizon. It caught us in the long axis, with the Tower jutting up in front of our feet. The same view we had lying there together, but with us in it. The picture is blown up and hangs on the wall of our dining room. It's right next to the same picture from our first anniversary. And from our fifth. Next installment is at ten.

Just the other day Steph said, "You know, you were right, I'll never forget that party."

My wife, Stephanie, is phenomenal. This is clearly obvious to everyone who knows her and substantially backed up by the fact that she can handle me at will.

I'm glad I didn't meet her when I was young because it would have been wasted. I would have wasted it with my naïve, youthful inability to know that people like this don't come along every day.

I can't help but mention my own realization when I write this. I was a wreck when I got divorced. I thought love was a farce. I thought it was just something to write songs and poems about, but in real life, it was a recipe for disaster. You were just going to get burned. I had trusted Jane with everything, and the carpet was pulled out from under me.

Little did I know, this was the very place I had to go to really find my true soul. Something started to happen to me in the depths of my own emotional torture chamber. I stopped focusing so much on *why*. Why was there so much suffering? Why was I so hurt and lonely? Why am I so worried about me, especially in the face of what I see? Slowly I began to see life differently. I began to take in, I mean really take in, the things around me that meant the most: my kids, my family, my friends. I stopped worrying about the *why*. I took the time to breathe, and it felt good. I had been so worried about where I was going that I forgot to enjoy just going.

As I mentioned, Stephanie's a firefighter-paramedic. She rotates on a crazy schedule, on forty-eight hours then off for ninety-six. So quite regularly, I'm left to my own devices. Basically, a bachelor two out of every six days.

The other night she called while she was at the firehouse. She was telling me about a call and firehouse politics and how she couldn't wait to get home the next day. That was all fine and well, but I kept trying to get off the phone. Subtle ploys at first, the things every guy is good at, but then it became more overt.

"Why do you want to get off the phone so bad?" she finally said, a bit irritated.

"*The Notebook*." I said it flatly, with a bit of embarrassment, but also a bit of resolve. *The Notebook* was on TV. I'm not a fan of the scenes with the *Rockford Files* guy and whoever the older lady is, but when the couple is young, in love, Ryan Gosling–style. . . . They had me at hello. I know that's a different movie, but you get the point.

You may be wondering why a guy like me likes *The Notebook*. Or why I'm even admitting it.

I like it for the moment of clarity.

When I sense from the actors what I feel about my wife and my family. I have trouble putting it into words so maybe you should just watch it. If I come home from work, and *The Notebook* is on, then I'm watching. Of course, some movies might trump it, like *Shawshank*, or *Bagger Vance*, but otherwise, *The Notebook* wins.

The moment of clarity, when I feel really, really, in love with Steph. The moment I let go of all the petty things that come between us and create distance in our relationship. When I truly feel what makes us a brilliant couple. I wish I could conjure these feelings at will, but I can't. I think it is the distraction of normal life. Especially when she is ticking me off. That's why I need *The Notebook*.

Can I ask for a time-out? Yes, I'm going on a tangent again. I want to talk about physics.

When I learned about physics in high school and college, I struggled over the equations of prediction and explanation. Physics was a science that explained the world. It explained the way things worked, and how one thing interacted with another. And even though I grappled with the math, it seemed to make sense and follow rules. I could predict the flight of a spaceship intercepting the path of an asteroid careening toward Earth, or calculate the pull of the electromagnetic force from one object to another.

But so much seems different now. Those finite things that I used to calculate don't seem like they are enough. There is so much more to this universe. Black holes, quantum mechanics, parallel universes, and extra dimensions. Forget about flight paths and electricity; now I have to think about strings, quanta, and dark matter.

I feel like this is similar to my life. I used to think things were predictable, explainable, that one event followed another, with rhyme and reason. But so much of what I've seen and experienced would indicate the opposite.

It's all so confusing.

And we don't even know what we are looking for. It's like my son on his physics homework: *To be honest, I don't even know what I'm doing here.*

But there is something. It is hidden, just out of view.

My wife was born in 1981. The same year I was really into "Tainted Love" by Soft Cell and the space shuttle *Columbia*. There is a bit of an age gap there. I graduated from med school when she graduated from high school, which I think is pretty cool.

We apparently like to get into arguments. Usually over stupid stuff. We rarely fight about things of relevance, but that would track with the majority of things I spend my life worried about.

When we have these dumb arguments, my wife and I have come up with a plan. It involves tequila.

Here's how it works. No, not the tequila. I learned about how that works not only in med school, but also on a trip to Mexico. Rather, I'm talking about the tequila as a tool. Whenever we get into a fight, regardless of who started it, either one of us can call a time-out. We don't actually say *time-out* and do quotes with our fingers or anything. The one calling the time-out merely stops talking, walks over to the liquor cabinet, and pours two shots of tequila. No one can argue until the drink is complete. I've even brought her tequila in the shower, in the morning, around 10:00 a.m. Because it's a time-out. It can happen at any time.

The whole idea might seem a little crazy and alcoholic, but it isn't. It is a simplistic intervention that works. Here's why.

Deep down I know I love her, and deep down she loves me. We get so caught up in the moment, focus on petty things, that we just forget the deep truth. I forget the things I feel in the moment of clarity when I'm watching *The Notebook*. The tequila acts as a break, a reboot and reset. It is ridiculous to have to take a shot of tequila in the middle of an argument, especially at 10:00 a.m., in the shower. The tequila is harsh, like someone slaps you in the face to snap you out of it. So when you take the shot, it freezes time and then resets. Big forward, small back.

I have spent my life trying to calculate an equation. I gripped on to life like I was working out a Newtonian problem. Plan, predict, follow through. That's how I thought it should work. But life isn't like that. It's more like dark matter. It's more like tequila.

A moment of clarity. A *Notebook* moment. A kiss on the bridge. Or even more profound, a kiss in the ICU. A kiss laced with life, death, and uncertainty.

PART V

HEROES

"One More Light" Linkin Park

If the joke included references to Catholics, or Irishmen, or best of all Catholic Irishmen, it was his favorite joke." Cathy Mayer laughed as she said it. "From Day One, he was gregarious, noisy, cheerful, and rambunctious."

Cathy Mayer was the program director for Flight for Life. She had taken the podium after the priest had finished Mass.

In an email to Mayer, Mahany had written, "It will be a small way that I can remain connected to the one program that I love. You are and always will be held very close in my heart. Please allow me to remain a tiny part of Flight for Life."

Finishing her eulogy, Cathy began to cry. "Well, Patrick, you did have to give that up and we have to give you up, far too suddenly and far too soon, but you are never a tiny piece of Flight for Life. You were close to the heart and the soul of our program."

Cathy sat, and three more family members stood, Pat's granddaughter flanked by his two grandsons.

"He was a wild man with a heart of gold." Nordine smiled as she said it.

She recalled catching her ski tip while going up A-Basin's Pallavicini lift with her Grandpa Pat: "I couldn't ride up the lift like that. He jumped with me. Like I said, he never let me go. I loved him dearly." Noticeably struggling, she finished, "And now it's our turn to never let him go."

The NTSB released their investigation of the crash. They determined that the probable cause of the accident was the "(1) preflight hydraulic check, which depleted hydraulic pressure in the tail rotor hydraulic circuit, and (2) lack of salient alerting to the pilot that hydraulic pressure was not restored before takeoff. Such alerting might have cured the pilot to his failure to reset the yaw servo hydraulic switch to its correct position during the preflight hydraulic check, which resulted in the lack of hydraulic boost to the pedal controls, high pedal forces, and a subsequent loss of control after takeoff."

The NTSB went on to report that the crash was survivable. However, because the helicopter was not equipped with a crash-resistant fuel system, the post-crash fire contributed to the lethality of the event. The fuel tank in the AStar is a fabric shell rather than reinforced metal. The crash caused fuel to leak out of the tank, contributing to the fire. Nomex flight suits protect you from a flash, not from sustained fire.

The color guard continued to stand at attention at either side of the stage. The priest and choir stood motionless in the back corner of the stage, off behind the coffin.

Pat's son took the podium. He was a strapping soldier. His uniform was already highly decorated, and he wore his beret low over his eyebrows with the fold off to the side, as is customary. He's also a helicopter pilot, like his father before him. *Star Wars* reference intended.

"Of course, I'm very proud," Pat had said of his son in a recent interview.

Flying a Blackhawk, Ryan Mahany had rescued two downed pilots who had crashed in Afghanistan in the Tora Bora region. An Apache helicopter was shot down during the rescue mission, and Ryan returned to rescue those two pilots as well. For the double rescue, Ryan was awarded the Air Medal for valor.

Ryan took the stage and began to speak.

"It is a fact that from the moment Dad died until this very moment today, he has never been alone. For all that, my family—my family is in your debt forever."

Ryan mentioned that he was getting ready for another deployment and that he hoped he could serve his men as well as his father had his. The speech was impossible to deliver. His wife, knowing his utter despair, stood up and moved behind him. Maybe she has superpowers too, like my wife.

He continued, determined.

"As this week has gone by and I've been speaking to a lot of Dad's friends, I am struck by the fact that many of you . . . know a lot about me . . . and my life." Both Ryan and the crowd laughed. "Many of you have touched my soul by telling me how proud he was of me." He struggled to continue. "But let me tell you this. . . ." Again, a pause and a sniffle. His wife stood steadfast. The crowd had become totally silent. "I was more proud of *him*." His voice popped as he said it. "And I will spend the rest of my life honoring his memory."

Big forward, small back. The moment extended.

"My father was my hero, and his untimely departure, it did crush my soul." The struggle was more forceful now. The grip of his wife deepened. "I'm angry he's gone. . . ." There was more wavering. "But I do cherish the memories that I have."

He continued to push through, grinding his teeth and squeezing the lectern. I could see his jaw flex. He plodded on, like a good soldier.

I felt the emotion. It was raw and unfiltered. My wife squeezed my hand harder as he struggled to complete his sentences.

It was uncomfortable because it was so real, so true. He admitted he was angry. This was refreshing. These weren't words from a priest. This was a son mourning the loss of his father.

He concluded by saying that his father would want this to be "a celebration of life."

I've heard that before at funerals, and I have to say that in the moment, it didn't feel like a celebration.

COCKTAIL PARTY

"Demons" Imagine Dragons

I was at a cocktail party not too long ago. My wife was socializing with some friends. She's good at it. Not me. I'd rather find a quiet corner to hide away with a friend or roam around by myself, taking in the view, people-watching. A lot of times people are better to watch than to talk to.

But at a cocktail party sometimes it's unavoidable. You have to talk. Especially when your wife asks you to be social. I was stuck in this group of people I didn't know, each of them seemingly wanting to talk more than the last.

In a break from them trying to one-up each other with their tales of impacted wisdom teeth, a woman asked me what I did. I told her I was an ER doctor. My mentor used to hate when we'd say *ER doctor*. He was a stickler for detail, and he would always say, "Can you only do your job in an emergency room? No, you can do your job anywhere. You're an expert in emergency medicine, not just an emergency room doctor." He also made us use a click pen. Taking a cap off a pen and putting it back on took too long. If you added up all the time you spent in this useless task over the course of an ER shift, you'd see that it cost you some real time. Hence, we all used click pens. I still use a click pen.

When asked what I do, what he'd wanted me to say was that I was an emergency medicine physician. That seemed like a lot of syllables.

I answered, "ER doc."

That piqued her interest. "That's cool!"

"Yeah," I replied. I was eyeing my escape route.

"Hey, have you ever seen anyone die?"

I hesitated and took a drink of my beer.

"Yeah, I've seen someone die."

"Oh, wow. That's crazy! How often?" she said, interrupting our conversation to smile and wave emphatically to a friend across the room. "Like, a few times?" she prodded.

"Yeah, something like that," I said, still planning my exit.

"What's the worst thing"—she became excited—"I mean. the most awful thing you've ever seen?" She took another gulp of her white wine.

You know what I said?

Nothing.

I said nothing.

Another woman standing in our little group jumped in. "I was in the ER once. This guy in the room next to me came in with blood all over his face. I think he got hit with a bottle or something. I had chest pain. The doctor didn't know what the hell he was doing because he sent me home and said I'd be fine. He said it wasn't a heart attack.

Said something was wrong with my lung or something. Clueless."

"What happened? Were you OK?" the dead-question lady asked.

"Oh, I'm fine. It just went away."

I may seem distracted at times. My kids and wife would probably say it happens a little more often than I'd care to admit. It's not that I can't focus; just the opposite. I get so caught up in what I'm thinking about that I often turn off the rest of the world. I can completely home in on a thought or task. My mom would attest to this from all the times she had to yell at me while I was watching a TV show, working on a model, or reading while growing up.

I'm sure it's frustrating to my kids—and to my mom (and to my wife), but it can be totally beneficial in a chaotic place like the ER. The ability to focus on something, when things are going apeshit all around you, has clear advantages.

At the cocktail party, that lady asking me the dead questions and the others in our small group—they probably thought I was distracted or aloof. And I was. To them. I was lost in thought. When she asked me if I had seen someone die, I thought of people actually dying.

I thought of Steve and Joss.

I thought of the guy in the helicopter.

I thought of the kid, his eyes dead, empty, looking nowhere into space.

I was narrowing down my answers to my Top 10 list, like Letterman. I was replaying it in my mind, video clips, but with emotion and true content. My distraction was only perceived on the outside, but internally, there was fierce focus. Thoughts that aren't escapable. Thoughts that pull me into the black hole.

But this, somehow, through a strange stream of consciousness, caused me to think about my kids. And then my wife.

I looked for her across the room, through the group of ladies standing in front of me. I caught a glimpse, in profile, but I could see her talking and laughing. She's always the life of the party.

I felt time. It slowed in the moment. Big forward, small back. Slow motion, one, because of the woman in front of me asking dead questions, and two, because of that image of my wife.

My life flashed in front of me. Not big moments like you would think. Not cliché. I thought about inconsequential things. One after another. My wife was in line at the grocery store, then chasing our dog in the yard, then changing a diaper. All of these moments, small and fleeting, brought me into her.

I saw her standing on the bridge in Paris. I saw the European sky behind her. The church steeple. The river with a small black-hulled boat floating below.

I was a man on fire. Time continued to move. The ladies at the cocktail party continued to talk. And my heart beat with time, big forward, small back, big forward, small back.

So much had culminated in this moment. Leaving the Academy, racing bikes, becoming a doctor, getting divorced. All things that seemed so monumental and at times insurmountable came together to give me this exact moment in space and time. In the beginning, you don't always see the end. I was in the moment.

I stared at my wife, until she finally looked my way and smiled. That perfect smile, where she is truly happy. When her upper lip pulls up and her nose wrinkles, just like her sister, so that I know it is real and not contrived or fake. Even though she was across the room, I knew what she knew, what we knew together: that we could run through a minefield or stroll through a garden, and either way, I would want to hold her hand with determination and passion, like it was a moment that might not last, like I was sitting at a funeral.

Here's the thing. I like losing myself in these "distractions." It's an escape to the timeless, a reflection into the knowing. It helps me feel alive. I'm not just brushing over stuff. I'm taking it in, even if the moment of knowledge and reflection hurts.

So much of my life has been wasted. I'm not talking about these moments at a cocktail party where I find myself staring at my wife. These may be when my mind is at its best. It's the hustle of my daily life that concerns me. My constant battle with the now. The running around frantically. My worrying life. I spend so much time vexed about what's next, how I get here or there, what I have to do today. Things get lost in the minutiae. I forget to look at the view. And this view is splendid.

I spend a lot of my life in the moment but not. If that makes any sense. I'm in the moment as far as the task at hand, but it's a manipulation rather than a feeling. What I want is an acceptance of the emotion. Resolution to live truly in the moment, the real moment, with depth. The smile that pulls in the upper lip and scrunches the nose so it is real. I want to be like that dog in the picture I mentioned earlier, the one with a distracted man. The dog is focused, doesn't care about the car, an airplane, a house, money. I want to live right now and experience all life has to offer.

I know, I experience, that everything can be taken away in a heartbeat. I know that at any given moment, everything that I hold most dear can be gone. It's fragile. With that knowledge, I can live a full life. I'm freed to live life because I have to accept the now and all the splendor that brings.

At the cocktail party all of these thoughts raced through my head as I stared past the woman and her drink, as I caught a glimpse of my wife chatting with her girl-friends. Talking about the inconsequential is fine; that's what you're supposed to talk about at a cocktail party. The latest movie, what Taylor Swift just did, the Kardashians, a new car. It's not for the depth of meaning. It's for con-versation. But people living and dying in the ER, the depth of real life and death? It is a vast story that isn't for cock-tail parties. The story isn't entertainment. It's a lesson in life. It's what lets me grow and breathe, be a great husband, strive to be the best father. It is all mine. It is mine and my wife's from across the room with that awesome smile. The story can't be used for anything less.

That's why I said nothing.

GSW

"Whiskey on My Breath" Love and Theft

Full *Trauma Activation, five minutes. Full Trauma Activation, five minutes.* I heard the paging system sound off while I was dealing with a belly pain in Room 5.

I walked out of the room to the front desk.

"Dr. McCollester says we need the OR." The tech delivered me the message.

"What do you mean? Where's Lock?" I said, a bit confused.

Dr. McCollester, Lock, is one of my partners, an ER doc in our practice. However, he wasn't working tonight.

The tech tried to clarify: "The paramedic said that Dr. McCollester is requesting the OR."

"For the trauma?" Still confused. "Is he on scene?" I said.

"I don't know," the tech answered, shrugging.

"Well, give me the info. What's the trauma?"

The tech was interrupted by the charge nurse: "GSW to the abdomen. They are coming emergent," she said.

"OK. And Lock is with them?"

"I don't know," she answered.

I walked into the trauma bay to prepare the room and get suited up. I pulled on the disposable yellow gown that keeps me from getting blood on my scrubs. As I slipped on a mask with a face shield, I thought about the possibilities. Likely, Lock was nearby when the guy got shot and decided to ride in with the ambulance. Or . . . Lock was the patient. But that would be pretty weird. Why would Lock be shot?

I went about my normal trauma setup. I turned on the video laryngoscope and pulled out an 8.0 ET tube, Macintosh #3, and bougie. The respiratory therapist was getting the BVM ready and hooking up suction.

Members of the trauma team started to arrive and check in. A trauma team activation is an ordeal, at least from a crowd control standpoint. Too many people for my liking. All the different departments in the hospital that are relevant to a trauma show up to the ER. X-ray, CT, and lab techs, representatives from the blood bank, OR staff and charge nurse, registration, primary nurse, secondary nurse, trauma surgeon, and more than a handful of others all congregate in the room or hallway.

The hardest part of a full trauma resuscitation isn't what you think. It's not the patient. It's controlling all these people. It becomes loud and sometimes unruly. They know they are supposed to be quiet, but when you put that many people together, with the added excitement of a full trauma arriving, things can escalate quickly. Small noises and quiet talking often build, like they do when you're in a restaurant with a large dinner party. The sound in the trauma bay ramps up, not because people are trying to be loud, but because of the number of people giddy with doing their job. Keeping a handle on the room is key.

The charge nurse came up to me again and asked, "What's the deal with Lock?" She added, "Is he the patient?"

"*Is* he the patient?" I said back.

I walked out of the room over to the tech's desk. I asked Lana, who had taken the call, "Is Lock with them, or is he the patient?"

"I don't know," she answered me, the same as the first time I asked.

Still puzzled, I headed back to the room. Slowly I heard the volume escalating. People were mumbling about the GSW (gunshot wound) and Lock.

"Hey all, listen up," I said firmly, speaking to the whole trauma room and breaking the increasing drone of noise in the room.

"I'm not sure if Dr. McCollester is with the patient or *is* the patient. But here's the deal."

The room was quiet and everyone was looking at me.

"Everyone try to be quiet. Just do your normal job. If it is Lock, it's going to get hectic so pay attention and listen to me."

Dr. Kyle Marthaller walked up, and I gave him the quick rundown. Trauma surgeons and ER docs work together on trauma activations. "Shit," he said calmly.

Just then the registration lady said the ambulance had pulled into the bay.

Forty-five seconds passed.

The doors slid open with a *swoosh*. It *was* hectic, that was obvious. Lots of people, EMS and firefighters, were already attending to Lock. He *was* the patient.

The gurney turned the corner into the trauma bay.

"This is Dr. McCollester. He was shot one time at close range. The bullet went through his arm and into his abdomen. I couldn't get a pressure at first, but his last BP was normal."

Six people moved around the bedside to get a grip on the sheet to slide him over to the hospital bed. Lock is a big, buff dude. It was a bit tricky because he was lying on his left side in the fetal position. He was gutturally yelling in pain. Someone was holding the dressing on his right arm.

The paramedic continued, "We found him on scene with two injuries, his arm and his abdomen. He has been awake and alert. A little hypotensive before getting fluid."

Just then he was interrupted by Lock: "It took out my ulnar nerve and . . ." He paused and contorted his entire body into a tighter fetal ball. "Ahhhrrrrhhh."

I started my exam, same as always. "Hey, Lock," I said, not waiting for an answer.

Airway. Breathing. Circulation.

"HEY, LOCK." I was still trying to get his attention. He was totally distracted by the pain.

The volume steadily increased. Not only was Lock yelling, but the chatter had crescendoed into a loud hum.

"Quiet down," I said loudly. "Quiet down!" I said again, even louder.

I gave it a second and people quieted. Lock still yelled.

"Get me a set of vitals and a second IV."

I focused on Lock.

"Hey, man. Listen to me. I need to check you out."

He growled a bit louder. But at least I could tell his airway was open.

"Hey, man, are you breathing OK?" I asked. I tried to uncoil him so I could get a look at his chest. The way he was crumpled up, I couldn't really see anything on his anterior chest or abdomen. There was a lot of blood smeared over his arm, hand, abdomen, and chest.

He seemed to move good air, but he had a rapid respiratory rate.

Either he didn't hear me or he was too distracted. Again, he didn't answer, just growled.

"Lock, look at me. Help me out. You know the deal. I need to check you out." I said it looking directly into his eyes.

"Yeaaahhh," he yelled. He had equal chest rise.

I was holding on to his wrist to check his pulse. I tried not to manipulate his arm, but he writhed in pain. His pulse was quick but strong. It also meant the GSW hadn't totally taken out his vascular structure.

"Lock, wiggle your fingers and toes." It's my standard statement to check D: Disability.

"Arrrrhhhhaaaa." Lock continued to yell.

"How much fentanyl did you give him?" I asked the medic, who was still standing in the room.

"One hundred," he responded.

"OK, let's give him another 150 mikes of fentanyl." I looked directly at the nurse with the drug box.

Bullets are tricky. I had been taught never to write "entrance wound" or "exit wound" on the chart. That is making too much of an assumption. You can take that with a grain of salt if the guy is telling you he got shot in the stomach. Chances are he probably got shot in the stomach. The point is that you just never know where a bullet goes. Once inside the body it can go up, down, right, or left.

I had a patient once who was shot in the neck. The bullet hit his cervical spine and then traveled all the way down to his abdomen. No exit wound. No obvious wound of any sort but his neck. It was tricky because his airway was stabilized, and the bleeding from his neck wound on the surface was controlled, but he was spiraling out of control. Turned out he was bleeding into his abdomen. He subsequently arrested. The thoracotomy revealed all the blood in his belly. The thoracotomy should have happened sooner, but there was no way to know with his initial presentation. An ultrasound would have helped, but at the time I didn't routinely US the belly with a neck wound.

Lock gave a pretty good, focused description when he did talk. "It took out my ulnar . . . arrrrhhhh, nerve . . . arrghhh, and it's in my abdomen." But I was still a little unclear as to the exact situation.

Was he shot once or twice?

Was he mugged or robbed?

Was this just a stray bullet?

The questions weren't a distraction. It was more that my brain was just trying to grasp the situation. To solve the puzzle to ensure that I wasn't missing anything.

I tried to ask Lock some more questions, but he was unable to respond. Too much pain. Too much struggle. He continued to contort into the fetal position. I still couldn't get a look at his abdomen or side.

"Lock, I'm going to give you some pain medicine. You got to help me out. I've got to take a look at you."

He continued to groan. The room was getting loud again.

I assessed the best I could, but after another thirty seconds I realized this wasn't going to work. I always teach medics that they need to be good at three things in order to do their job well:

1. Clinical Knowledge
2. Technical Skill
3. Scene Control

I was experiencing a scene control issue. Lock was in so much pain I couldn't assess him. This was adding to the hectic nature of a critical patient.

"Hey, man, I need to get a look at you. Lock, I'm going to RSI you. I'm going to put you to sleep. OK?" I didn't really wait for his response before I continued. "Let's RSI," I said, turning to the nurse with the medications.

Another nurse interrupted, "You want blood?"

"Yeah, hang it up."

I looked back to Lock. I had expected him to defy my request. I had expected him to refuse the RSI. I don't know any ER doc who is keen on having one of his partners RSI him. But he didn't object. In fact, he seemed to welcome it.

I mentioned this earlier. RSI is a technique of sedating a patient, paralyzing them, and then placing a breathing tube. It happens rapidly and in sequence, hence the name. It's a legit intervention. Meaning, it is serious.

The paralysis is exactly what it sounds like. A patient is unable to move. They can't even breathe. When a doc performs RSI, he is taking the patient's life into his own hands. I always say that when you RSI a patient you are killing them and then bringing them back to life. Lock would know all this. He would know that if something went wrong, he could die. If I couldn't get an airway on Lock, I would kill him.

"OK, do it. Just do it." His answer was calm, without volume. It was the clearest answer I had gotten from Lock since he arrived.

I was standing right next to Dr. Marthaller, the trauma surgeon. We looked at each other briefly. I might be reading into it, but I feel like he gave me a look, only for an instant, that said, *Holy shit, you're going to tube Lock.*

I interrupted the commotion once again.

"Draw up 160 of ketamine and 120 of succs," I said, looking at the nurse.

"Got it. 160 milligrams of ketamine and 120 milligrams of succinylcholine," she repeated.

Ketamine is Special K. It's a dissociative agent. It separates the patient from reality. That's why it's a street drug as well. It also has the properties of treating pain and anxiety. All things I wanted for Lock. Additionally, it didn't drop blood pressure as much as other agents, like etomidate, so it was ideal in trauma.

Succinylcholine, succs, is a depolarizing paralyzing agent. It rapidly relaxes the patient so the endotracheal tube can be placed more readily. It also prevents the patient from vomiting during the procedure. Vomiting is a big risk because, unlike people undergoing elective surgery, where you are instructed not to eat or drink after midnight, emergency patients may have just eaten a big meal.

I organized my intubation equipment and took a deep breath. Honestly, I didn't feel extra-nervous, but I did think about the fact that I was about to intubate a friend. It was an unemotional thought, though. It was a drastic difference from my first night in the ICU during residency, when I tried to control my breathing as my leg bounced out of control. I was steady and calm. Detached but present. I'd never intubated a friend who also happened to be an ER doc. But there's a first time for everything.

On my order, the nurse pushed the ketamine. I leaned over Lock. "I'm going to take good care of you. I got you, man." Lock and I connected our gaze.

I waited briefly. I looked up to the nurse, nodded, and she pushed the succs. The room became calm. This was the quietest it had been since this all started. I didn't even have to ask for it. People understood the gravity of the situation. I paused and looked at my watch. Ten seconds. Big forward, small back. Twenty seconds. Thirty seconds. Big forward, small back. Thirty-five seconds went by, and I saw Lock's muscles start to "fasciculate," the medical term for *twitch*. This is why it is called a depolarizing paralytic. It depolarizes the cells first, causing the movement or twitching, and then paralyzes them.

On cue, the groaning and writhing stopped. Lock lay calmly.

I slowly scissored his mouth open and slid in the intubating blade. It was a straightforward view on my video laryngoscope. I progressively moved down his airway, from the oral pharynx, the uvula, the posterior pharynx, and the tip of the epiglottis, into the vallecula, and finally to a clear view of the vocal cords. With my right hand, I applied forward pressure to the endotracheal tube and without hang-up, slipped it through paralyzed cords.

I removed my blade and inflated the tube cuff balloon.

Misting and capnography looked good. Normal breath sounds with bagging.

The room started to move again. I think everyone had been holding their breath when I placed the tube. Everyone, including Lock, could breathe again. The respiratory therapist (RT) started to ventilate with the BVM. I spoke with the RT about ventilator settings.

The staff organized the vent, monitor, and IV, and all the cords and tubing that went along with them. We were off to the CT scanner. Some surgeons would go directly to the OR, but since he was hemodynamically stable, Dr. Marthaller wanted a better idea of where the bullet was and what damage it caused.

Lock's arm was mangled, but that wasn't our immediate concern. The bleeding from the wound seemed to be controlled. He appeared to have a nerve injury, but that wasn't going to kill him. Right now, we were intent on looking at where the bullet was sitting and what damage had occurred as the shock wave from the penetration tore at the tissue.

"I'm going upstairs to scrub in," Dr. Marthaller said. I stayed with Lock until the end of the scan, and then we wheeled him up to the OR.

I returned to the ED (the Emergency Department) and paged ortho. The first guy on call didn't want to come in to see him because he wasn't on for "hand." I explained that he was shot in the forearm, not the hand. I also told him it was Lock. The ortho doc had worked here for years. We all knew each other, but that didn't sway him. He wouldn't come in. I would love to write his name here, but I'll restrain myself.

I called the second ortho on call, specifically for hand. Again, I explained the injury, and then, I explained that it was Lock. He said that it wasn't his responsibility. I should talk to the "general orthopedist." He was only on for hand. I would also love to write his name here.

You got to be fucking kidding me.

I know I italicized it like I was thinking it, but I may have said it out loud.

I called a third ortho doc. I didn't want to call the number-one guy on call back to argue, because fuck him. So I called a guy who I knew would help. Dr. Jackson called back promptly. I told him the situation. "I'm on my way in."

Dr. Jackson arrived at the ER, and we reviewed the situation. "Damn," was all he said, then went upstairs to the OR.

I walked back to the trauma room and saw the EVS (Environmental Services) team cleaning up. A lone nurse stood at the computer terminal, working on her charting. Everyone else had left.

I still had a few hours left in my shift. I would have loved to call it a day, but people kept checking in. The ER didn't shut down. That's not what we do.

I finished my shift and signed out to the oncoming ER doc. After taking a minute to step outside and breathe the fresh air, I headed to the ICU to check on Lock. He was quiet, lying in bed, probably unaware that I was there. I just stood there, looking at a severely broken ER doc. A friend. I didn't say anything.

It was late when I finally got home. I tried to ninja up the stairs, but with every step the old house creaked. I came into our bedroom and pulled off my clothes, then turned on the shower. My wife makes fun of me because when I'm really tired or stressed, I just stand in the shower with my arms folded, motionless, water hitting me in the back of the neck. I assumed the position.

I finally stepped out and quietly dressed. I grabbed the top T-shirt in my closet and an old pair of sweatpants. I couldn't see because the lights were off, but I could tell from the thin worn-out feeling of the cotton shirt that it was one of my favorites. My wife roused in bed and said, "Everything OK? Did you have a bad shift?"

"Yeah."

She knew me well enough not to ask. I walked over and kissed her on the head. I took a moment so I could take in the smell. Then I headed back downstairs.

Dinner was waiting. And, more importantly, a whiskey.

MASTER OF THE UNIVERSE

"Voodoo Chile (Slight Return)" Jimi Hendrix

I'll admit this simple conclusion: if it were all up to me I would have blown it. If I were master of my universe, I would have missed out on the best things in my life. In the middle of trying to hold on so tight, trying to align everything perfectly, I wouldn't have been able to get out of my own way.

I was at a bar with friends, and we were playing life-size Jenga. The blocks were cut out of two-by-fours. We took turns stacking one block on the other to see how high we could get the tower. OK, technically not really Jenga, but the opposite—building up piece by piece instead of taking it down. We got it pretty high. At one point I was on the shoulders of a six-three firefighter trying to put on the next block. It probably comes as no surprise that it might not have been the best idea. The whole tower toppled over, nearly taking both of us out. Don't worry, the beer broke my fall.

As you may have noted, I'm pretty much obsessed with physics, quantum physics specifically. Parallel universes are a close second. My wife loves talking about it at dinner. Not.

Sometimes when things are going poorly, when things aren't going the way I think they should, not going according to *my* plan, I switch into physicist mode. I move to the mode of parallel universes. I try to envision another version of me. The version where I see things going perfectly.

Infinity is a big number. My dad would ridicule me for writing a sentence of such understatement. Infinity *is hard* to grasp. If the universe were infinite—which is up for debate, but if we assume, for the sake of argument, that it is—then any constellation of events that brought me to this exact place at this exact time, no matter the odds against it, could also be occurring exactly the same way somewhere else.

In fact, if we accept an infinite universe, then there are infinite similar circumstances bringing a replica of me to this unique situation. There is another place where this finite (yes, finite, not infinite) set of circumstances occurred from the beginning of time until now to make me. All the pieces fell perfectly into place. Every atom zigged instead of zagged, at every conceivable point and moment, to produce an impeccable replica of me, somewhere in the far stretches of the infinite universe. Even more impressive, in the infinite universe, there would be an infinite number of strict replicas of me, right up to this moment. Infinite me's.

Right now, one of these versions of me is sitting and typing these very words at a computer. But also, right now, there is another version of me writing *better* words than these, making a better version of this very book. What if I could somehow access one of those versions? Any of those versions? Could I just jump from soul to soul? I mean, it is me we're talking about here.

Every time something sucked, I could magically, scientifically, jump into another me. I could avoid all the moments that are less than tolerable.

On the surface that sounds sweet. Where's that wormhole? I want to jump through, always warping myself to the me that is making the better, wiser decision, avoiding all the pitfalls.

There would never be a moment of indecision when taking care of a patient, or setting a rule for my kids, or talking back to my wife. Because I could essentially have a do-over. I could get out of any fix. I'm not following God's rules anymore. Like I said before, I'd run things differently, so this is perfect.

But what if I could do that, jump through the wormhole to a different me? A better me. If I lean back in my chair, close my eyes, and think about it, things start to get fuzzy. Philosophy fuzzy. Who-is-the-owner-of-the-*Sea-Squirrel* fuzzy. What would my life be like—jumping from me to me?

Well, for starters, I think it would be lame.

Avoiding the suck would make my life suck.

Bet you didn't see that coming. I'm telling you, I really did lean back, close my eyes, and think about this . . . for a while. Try it. It might surprise you.

You've heard the story of the kid that snuck some candy from the kitchen pantry? The parents, annoyed by the theft and the dishonesty, lock the ne'er-do-well kid in the closet with all the chocolates, the entire Costco bag. He's not allowed to come out until the bag is completely finished. Most kids think this is a pretty awesome punishment—a closet, a bag of chocolates, and no parental guidance. But then things turn ugly. After an hour in the dark closet with a half-eaten bag and a big belly ache, the lesson starts to become clear. What started as a punishment straight from heaven turned into torture. The good chocolate became bad chocolate. Good becomes bad. Cool, not so cool.

Maybe something like the kid in the closet would happen to me if I jumped from soul to soul. Not that I'd get a bellyache, but maybe I'd start to become bored with the whole thing, and I hate being bored.

Good events, one after the other, on and on indefinitely, maybe wouldn't be as fantastic as I initially thought. If a good event was the norm, time after time, over and over, maybe it wouldn't be good. It would become kind of a defective existence.

The key here is that I need the backdrop to enjoy all the things I really treasure. How do I know how to feel true love for my wife if I've never felt the sting of loss?

I'm not saying that Joss or Steve should be thankful for what they went through. Or that the mom from Room 11 had some redemption. No way would I ever say that. I don't know if there is redemption from that. Maybe you're just done when something like that happens.

Maybe sometimes things are just shitty.

I don't like bad times any more than the next guy. Defense mechanism or no, I want to try to understand it. I do know that if the bad things in my life were taken away, there would be no way for me to feel what I feel in my best moments.

I come back to my discussions with my wife regarding faith, or my lack thereof, and to my anger with the feeling of loss and poor control. Every day that I question, I feel my faith is a bit stronger. Each and every time I struggle through the thought processes, looking for rhyme and reason to this whole existence, it grows a little stronger. I think it is like working out. Each day in the gym is hard, but over time I become stronger, better.

I want the expanse, a rainbow from end to end. Double rainbow, even. There's no vehicle for that if my experience is limited. I have to pay the price to open the door to more. More living, feeling, experiencing—everything that makes me a human soul.

So maybe, in those moments when things seem to be going the opposite of good, I shouldn't feel so forced to escape. I'm thinking that I shouldn't try to stack the pieces together like a game of Jenga. Ultimately, Jenga is a game that you can't win. Someone loses, but no one really wins. Because you can just keep stacking the pieces higher and higher. Eventually they are going to fall. That is physics.

Jenga. That's what I feel like with life as a whole. Stretching to place the next block. Holding on for dear life, hoping the whole thing won't topple over. For so much of my life I had just been playing Jenga. I had been into the perceived status of my life. I don't mean status like driving a Ferrari compared to someone else's Yugo. I'm talking about the status of things that I put in front of everything. Being successful in my career, being the best on a particular project, getting published, receiving honors on a rotation.

It was all importance I created in my head, part of a game I thought I could win. I had blocks precariously stacked one after the other—med school, residency, house, job, wife. I just continued to stack, thinking that more blocks were the key to my happiness. The higher, the better.

Patients never plan on coming to the ER. It's always unexpected. I didn't think that I'd fall off my six-three friend either. But, come on, that's just being naïve.

When I try to control every aspect of my life, I might be messing things up. I'm not understanding the setup, the rules. Holding on so tight might not be the answer. It might actually limit my participation.

The best hitters in baseball don't strangle the bat to death. They let the moment flow. That's what I need to do. I'm not saying to let go of the wheel completely. You do that when you're driving, or batting, and someone is going to get hurt. I'm just pointing out that I may need to loosen up my grip just enough to take a full swing. I need to relax, eat a chocolate or two. The best hitters, the moneymakers, only hit one out of every three. That's a lot of whiffs.

SURF

"The Search" NF

It was hot as hell. The water looked perfect. The patchy, deep blue sections were interspersed with sections mirroring the sun back into my face. There's something about getting into the ocean, a primal sense of evolution manifesting itself, from microorganisms all the way to my sweating, 70-percent-seawater body. I attached my leash and righted myself. Arching my back, I shaded my eyes attempting to get a read on the swell. I felt the sand squish between each toe, as I rocked back and forth trying to permanently install my footprint. Today I had decided on a six-eight fishtail. The waves weren't huge, and I hadn't surfed in a while—a good compromise between a sporty ride and an arm-burning paddle.

I grew up in Northern California. The water temp is fifty-five degrees year-round. I'm a bit of a cold wuss, so back home I wouldn't attempt to surf with anything thinner than a 5/3 suit, usually booties and gloves at a minimum. Today off the shore of Sayulita, Mexico, all I needed was a rash guard and board shorts to cover my albino-looking skin.

The water felt as good as it looked. After wading to knee depth I took the dive, gliding on top of the water, the popping sound of waves lapping against my board. I looked out and saw my buddies spread out like a platoon on patrol.

Man, I was out of shape, at least for surfing. All that paddling had really taken it out of me. I sat up, straddling my board, and shook my arms. They felt waterlogged and flimsy. My buddy looked over laughing. Most of the guys were already hitting it. It had taken me a bit longer to clear the break. Seems I timed it "just right" and hit every wave at the moment it was breaking.

I liked where I was sitting. There are two "safe" spots surfing: the shore and just outside the break. I collected myself as I watched the platoon's heads bob up and down as the swell moved through. Now you see them, now you don't. The rhythm of the waves was mesmerizing. I felt the sun on my face and the water engulfing my legs from the knees down. I wanted to sit here forever.

I paddled forward a bit, not with total confidence. I saw a new set off in the distance. If I wanted to ride I was going to have to move in. I pulled up a few feet from my buddy.

"It's good," he said, looking back over his shoulder.

"It's big," I said. Not sure if I meant, *Yeah, it's good and big, and that's good,* or *Yeah, it's good and big, and that's bad.*

My friend leaned forward and started paddling with some meaning off to his right. I saw it also. The water was pulling under nicely. Off a bit, I could see the front of the wave forming. Probably a four-five footer. Keep in mind that waves are measured from the backside. The measurement doesn't include all the water that is pulled up underneath on the front side. A four-five-foot wave might not sound like much if you don't surf or if you've watched big wave riders, but when you have my skill set and are in the trough, paddling to catch the wave, it looks freakin' huge.

I followed him and started to put my muscle into it, just to get up to speed. I paddled hard and heard the all-encompassing rush of the water start to build on either side. The power came under my board, and I began to lift. It felt like a conveyor belt moving slightly faster than I expected as it grabbed ahold of the sides of my board. I glanced off to my right, and my buddy was just starting to feel the sensation I had a few moments ago. I popped to a low crouch, and then, with only a moment to steady myself, I popped once again, this time to standing. I was launching forward, down the face of the wave with a smooth synchronicity that makes everything seem effortless and harmonious.

I cut up to the right. I was almost to the top of the wave before kicking my feet in the opposite direction to turn it back left. My buddy toppled over the front of his board in a magnificent display of aerobatics. The wave was all mine, free and clear. I could go wherever I wanted. The edge of my board dug in like it had some serious grip. The sensation was invigorating. It felt similar to carving a snowboard in Colorado powder. My smile must have looked something like the Joker from *Batman*. I was ecstatic. The ride lasted all of ten to fifteen seconds, but it felt like an entire vacation. I purposefully ended the ride with a digger to my right, standing up straight off my board and falling over onto my back as the wave burned out. I jumped back on top of my board and started to paddle out again. Now with more confidence.

I timed this paddle out better. I didn't seem to get hammered by every incoming wave. Maybe I just needed to loosen up a bit with a good ride. I splashed some salt-water into my face, and then shook my head hard like a dog. I could see the next set coming in. I moved to position myself.

I paddled forward and felt the water move around me. I could hear that the wave was ready to ride. The force came from under me like last time, and I quickly pulled myself to a squat. But this wave was way more forceful. I started down the face, this time too fast, too late, too everything that is not good. I tried to move my weight back, but my brain didn't compute the proprioceptive change with any-where near the needed efficiency as I started free-falling forward. The sharp front end of my board dove into the base of the wave, and like a medieval catapult, I felt myself launch forward.

There was a brief moment, an airborne moment, that I knew it was going to hurt a little. I pulled my knees up toward my chest and took a deep breath. I was going under. I hit with an insulting violence that was immediately fol-lowed by an almost bizarre calm. Then the wave, with no regret, yanked my board, which in turn yanked my leg. I flipped underwater. The undercurrent caught me, and I tumbled again. And again. I remained calm and partially limp, letting the wave do what it may. My feeble attempt at protecting my face didn't keep it from sliding along the sandy bottom. Now I had to try to remain calm more vig-orously. *Relax*, I told myself in a subconscious way. I could feel the oxygen being eaten up by all my cells. When I felt

I had waited an eternity, I kicked to the surface, eagerly preparing to breathe. It didn't come. As I bobbed up, I was immediately slammed by the next wave in the set.

I nearly drowned when I was young. I really did. And now it seemed it might be happening again. I grew up in the boondocks, Bones Road, as I mentioned before. When I was almost seven, I went on an adventure to a neighbor's pool. I don't mean this in any negative way, but they were straight-up hippies. The pool was just a big hole dug in the ground with a tarp suctioned to the edge by the water. I was on a raft. I remember slipping off and going under. I wasn't a good swimmer. I was, in fact, a bad swimmer. I had no business being in those hippies' pool, especially with no water wings or lifeguard. I tried for the surface but swam like I had a cinder block tied to my leg, kind of how my Doberman swims. I caught glimpses of sunlight shimmering at the surface, but I couldn't make it back to the raft.

The next thing I remember, I was lying on the side of the pool having my arms pulled back behind me, like this was the ideal medical treatment for a drowning seven-year-old. I was vomiting water. Again, I blacked out. I don't remember anything again, except glimpses of naked hippies scurrying about the edge of the pool, until I was sitting in a hospital bed at Sebastopol Memorial Hospital. I was now with my parents and my sister. As they came into my ER cubicle, I heard Missy, my sister, ask my dad, "Is Shannon going to die?"

Now in the Pacific, off the shore of Sayulita, I felt my lungs burn, begging for some oxygen. Strangely enough, without any panic, I contemplated that if I didn't get air soon, I'd die. I don't remember any actual panic looking up at the raft in that pool either. I was swimming hard, but not panicking. It was strange, both times.

At the last moment I got spit out like the ocean was hocking a loogie. I didn't know how it happened, and it certainly wasn't because of anything I had done, but I was on the surface, in the shallow water. I slowly lifted myself onto all fours, coughing, attempting to get the water out of the lower segments of my lungs.

I clutched my board, still hacking and breathing heavily. My ribs on the right were killing me. I had slammed onto the ocean floor, or my board, or something. I tried in vain to clean the sandy grit from my mouth by spitting. After a few seconds, regaining my wits, I stood up. I staggered like a grandpa crossing a river because my equilibrium was jacked. Seawater dripped from my face, ears, and eyes.

I slowly moved up onto the beach, getting out of range of any big rogue waves. The board dropped, and I flopped myself down on the sand. I lay there on my back, listening to the birds. So clear. The waves continued to methodically wash up on shore near my feet. I squinted one eye, kind of like a grimace, and let out an audible *ahhhhhhh*. I took a deep breath, holding it to the point of maximal inspiration because it stabbed me, and then let out another *ahhhhhhh*. This routine continued for God knows how long.

As I lay there and tried to recover, I watched the sky and listened to the rhythm of the ocean. I just got my assed kicked. But everything was clear. I could breathe. I was alive.

PART VI

LAST CALL

"Dare You to Move" Switchfoot

Pat's son returned to his seat, his wife by his side. There was an awkward pause as the funeral director and the priest shuffled about, figuring out what was supposed to happen next. More people, friends and a few family members, spoke. They offered some memories and then tried to give some personal bit of meaning to this whole messed-up situation.

I kept focus. But not on just one part of the funeral. Take it from an ER doc: polyfocus is a thing. I can concentrate on the procedure in front of me but also listen for beeps, phones, ambulance bay doors—all things that might need immediate attention.

I focused on the lake, glimmering so pure and blue in the distance, on Pat's son, stoic and strong in his uniform yet needing his wife to help give him support, and the coffin, with the white draping hung over the front, Pat's clean, undamaged helmet on the ground. I kept looking back and forth between these objects. Trying to make sense of the beauty, the emotion, and the loss all at once.

My focus on all these unique items was grounded. My wife, Stephanie, still recovering from the opening bagpipes and Ryan's speech, continued to squeeze my hand. I felt the strength and power of the grip, and I'm not talking about a weight lifting grip. I'm talking about the strength of what I felt for her. The same kind of feeling I had when I saw her across the room at the cocktail party. I felt the kind of love I had witnessed when Steve was rolled out of the hospital.

I focused on the clean silver helmet in front of the casket.

I thought about being strapped into the helicopter and feeling the sudden spin. Momentum pulling me toward the window. A drop and more spin, my stomach moving up to my throat like I was on a roller coaster.

I imagine a jaw-splitting impact. Similar to when I crashed on my bike. But way harder and more aggressive. The kind of impact that stuns your senses so you disconnect. I imagine the pop of flames. A moment of calm and then panic.

Suddenly I was back at the funeral looking at the clean, silver helmet.

It might be my ADHD talking here, but do you like whiskey? Yeah, we are moving off topic again. Whiskey is so intricate, complex, and full. I think the unique and solid taste helps build memories. You remember where you were and who you were with the first time you taste a special whiskey.

I love the process of distilling and aging. I got a crazy idea to make whiskey a few years back. Actually, for the sake of the book and my family, I got the idea of making fuel. You can legally make fuel for your car. You can also make essential oils. That doesn't sound quite right, so I'll go with the idea of making "fuel."

I had concocted a grand scheme for a distillery. I showed my wife what I had planned. She raised an eyebrow and with little to no thought immediately said no. "It looks like a meth lab." *Sweet, like Breaking Bad,* I thought. "No way," she said.

I think it looks nothing like a meth lab. It looks like a homemade still . . . OK, maybe a little like *Breaking Bad.* She didn't want any part of it, and I could tell this wasn't up for discussion.

That Christmas, just a few months later, I got an awesome present from Steph. It was a beautiful hammered-copper still. For essential oils . . . Fuel. For sure.

I've spent a lot of time figuring out how that thing works. But here is a summary. You take some sort of sugar-containing substance, like corn or wheat, and cook it a bit to release the inner ingredients. You add yeast, which eats the carbohydrates. This act of eating carbs creates alcohol as a by-product. You're left with a mix of unused glucose, yeast, and alcohol.

Take all this stuff, all mixed together and unpure, and put it in a still, *Breaking Bad*-style. If you cook it at the correct temperature, you get the alcohol to burn off more quickly than the other ingredients. Distillation. It is purification.

It is a time-consuming process overall. But that's what I need. A moment of pause, a moment of rest and clarity. I take a hodgepodge of ingredients, which is just like all the baggage that fills my daily life, and then I start to purify it. I distill everything I experience to get the end product, which is complex, robust, flavorful, and fantastic.

Maybe the analogy is a stretch. But this is just how I think, and it works for me. I always apply the stuff I like or understand to everything else, especially when the other stuff doesn't really make sense. Doctors are taught to think a certain way. I learned that from a lawyer. A buddy who was a corporate lawyer once told me on a chairlift at Vail, "I don't practice law, but I think like a lawyer. That's all law school is; it's a way to think."

I'd like to give myself credit (because doctors are always looking for ways to put down lawyers) and say that med school taught me not only a way to think, but also a whole shit ton of stuff about the human body and how to treat, diagnose, and manage disease. Way more than I would have learned in law school. But that's a bit of a tangent. I will say, though, that I get his point, and I agree.

Whiskey making, distilling, is what doctors do every day when trying to diagnosis unknown illnesses. We take a goulash of complaints, signs, and symptoms, apply it to some underlying databank of information and facts, and try to purify it down to a simple product or solution—a diagnosis. It's also like what I do in my life.

The priest stood at the front checking his notes one last time. The Mass was ending, and I could sense the service was nearly over.

He looked to the crowd and raised a hand. "May God lift up his soul from death, and give Patrick Mahany the best flight of his whole life."

He turned and yielded the stage to one last speaker. It was a dispatcher from Flight for Life.

John Resknic had been a dispatcher for Flight for Life for eight years. He took the podium for an unenviable task.

Last call.

This is where it got rough for me, like bagpipes for my wife.

It is customary for police, fire, and EMS to give a last call. This is a symbolic gesture of the dispatcher giving the final call to the deceased. All first responders live by the radio, directing them to distress, guiding them to others who need help. The radio is the tyrant and the savior.

The dispatcher quickly cleared his throat. I had no idea how he would get through this.

"Lifeguard 2, this is com center." He paused.

The pause was uncomfortable. Everyone was silent.

"Lifeguard 2, this is com center." Another pause.

This one a little bit longer. A little bit more uncomfortable.

I looked over at my wife and saw a tear rolling down her cheek from under her sunglasses. I had to look away from her. I couldn't take it. I looked out at the lake. So peaceful. So calm.

The clock moved, big forward, small back.

"Lifeguard 2, this is com center. . . . Patrick Mahany . . . you may stand down. End of watch."

Big forward, small back. Big forward, small back.

"Patrick Mahany . . . you may stand down. End of watch."

SAMUEL'S GRAVE

"So Alive" Goo Goo Dolls

I stopped by the little boy's grave last month. His name was Samuel. He was the little boy from the beginning of the book. Like I said earlier, there is a price. It never leaves me. The cemetery is at the north end of Boulder. There's a monument out front for fallen soldiers with a cannon and an American flag. When you drive in the gate you hang a hard right, then take a left at the first dirt intersection, to the second tree. That's where the grave is. I come here every so often. Not on an anniversary or anything, just when I feel the need to take a moment. Maybe I think it's like hitting the reset button.

The gravestone is typical, except for the dates. You wouldn't know it just by walking by, but if you actually read the dates, you'd quickly realize that the person here is ridiculously young. Just a little boy. The last time I stopped by, there was a die-cast Hot Wheels motorcycle, a pinwheel, and some dying flowers. The grave is well taken care of, but the flowers were still dead.

That's usually the case at cemeteries. Even when loved ones have the best intentions, when you find yourself walking through a cemetery, most of the flowers on graves are dead. Once in a while, you'll see a plot recently visited, flowers a day or two old, but that is more uncommon, because living things die. Some graves have fake flowers or plants, but they're just that: fake. Not real.

I don't think I have a problem with the dying flowers. I also think I have to apologize for the first chapter of this book. I might have told you an untruth. Funerals might not totally suck.

The first couple of times I came here I kept going through Samuel's case over and over, trying to figure out if there was something else I could have done, some other treatment or intervention that would have changed the outcome. I was kicking myself. What if I had recognized the pneumonia sooner? What if the parents had come in just twenty minutes earlier? What if the primary care physician's office wasn't completely booked when they tried to make an appointment? The *what ifs* can go on almost indefinitely. Armchair quarterbacking is easy, but in this case, also painful.

I sat down next to the grave and, well, just sat, nothing else. It must have been ten or fifteen minutes—recounting his face, his little fit body, his mother's look, her eyes. Her eyes never leave me. I was thinking about my kids. And Steph. I closed my own eyes and took in the moment. More appropriately, I was in the moment.

Sounds became a bit sharper. I could hear some birds off to my left, a prairie dog chirping not too far off behind me, and the low moan of a nearby busy street. The breeze blew to the east, and I felt it tickle my hair that had grown a bit longer than normal. Things seemed calm. Even the horrible memories of standing over Samuel, that monotone cardiac monitor and low-pitched oxygenation sound resonating in my memory, his mother's appropriate hate for me, and the staff's heads down. I found peace.

I lay back and opened my eyes. The clouds floated carelessly overhead, just like on the beach. Calm. I could hear the ocean in my mind. I felt that inside-out peace, and my heart slowed, like it was acknowledging the inevitable. There was no perseveration or anxiety. No more armchair. Just calm.

Sometimes the fear of something happening is worse than it actually happening. I was calm because I wasn't afraid of what might happen anymore. I had seen a kid actually die. In front of me. And he's not the only one, and if I keep working, he won't be the last. I accepted the truth. I didn't need a parallel universe or infinity. I didn't even want it.

I remembered the warning from Dr. Morgan, but I had only understood half the meaning, like the warning was bad. Sure, I lost my innocence, but with that loss came wisdom. I wanted the blue pill. Like I said before, building character sucks, especially when you're actually building character. The same is true for wisdom.

I have lost love, but only through that experience could I find my true love, a sonnet kind of love. I have seen kids die, and because of circling that black hole, I know how to love my own children.

I must have laid by Samuel's grave for a good thirty minutes. Caught in the moment, the dream, the reality. Then there was a car. It was pulling up to another grave nearby. I turned my head to the side and looked at all the little toys and knickknacks spread out over the groomed dirt. I breathed. The clouds continued to float overhead and the prairie dog continued to chirp. Life moved on and left the little boy behind. But then again it didn't. The clock moved big forward, small back. He was right here, telling me to loosen my grip.

ALL IN

"Good Life" OneRepublic

I didn't finish my surf adventure from the earlier chapter. I didn't die. Obviously. I lay there on the white sand, back wedging into the surface for an eternity, near as I could tell. Finally, I motivated myself to sit up. The sun was still shining like a billion bullets to my retinas. I was able to squint through it and see how the other guys were faring. Parker took a spectacular digger, a nosedive similar to what I had done. Joel cut on the break to the left and rode it in all the way to the whitewash. A couple of the other guys just continued to bob at the edge of the break. Maybe they were thinking they didn't want to die. Maybe they were just reading the swell. I wasn't sure. I worried they were floating out there, taking a time-out, just to wonder if I was a wuss because I was lying on the beach so damn long.

Ever since leaving the Academy, I had changed. I didn't want to lose control; I didn't want to fail. I certainly didn't want to quit. But in the end, I've come to know that failing or not, winning or losing, isn't really what it's all about—contrary to what Nike, Reebok, and Adidas might say. And I will tell you, quitting is not an option either. Appropriately or not, Winston Churchill has been credited with saying, *If you're going through hell, keep going.* It's a totally valid statement.

It isn't about my plan or my opinion. My thoughts on the matter are only that: mine. Nothing more or less. I have come to understand, to realize, that no matter how hard I try to control things, it is nothing more than a wringing of the hands. It's squeezing the bat too tight. The true adventure, the true possibility, is not really knowing what is next. True adventure is an autorotation, in control and out of control at the same moment.

I started this book by saying I was someone different. Someone my family wouldn't recognize. I said that I was always guarded, too guarded. And if you made it this far, we've come on a journey together. So I thank you for that.

I had no idea what I was getting into when I started to write *Fragile.* It is a scary proposition, writing. I should rephrase. Writing about something that is real, that requires you to search your core, is terrifying. I don't like to talk to people at a cocktail party, but here I am spewing my guts to whoever might pick up my book.

But *I* needed to write *Fragile.* I needed to try to make some sense of all of this craziness. I needed to somehow make amends with God. Grace is a big deal. I needed to accept that grace. But I also needed to give it. I'm not even sure if you can give grace to God, but I'm going with it.

I'm going out on a limb here, but there is an extremely high probability that everything won't go exactly the way I planned. Winning and losing are things that can happen when I'm in a soccer match or rolling jiujitsu. It just isn't what happens in life.

I sat in the sand, hand shielding my eyes, watching the beautiful blue ocean turn to white as it approached the shore. I hadn't moved, yet. I just sat, waiting.

Then it hit me. I had a revelation. I was only a wuss if I didn't try to ride again. If I let the fear of the slam and drowning keep me out of the water, then what they were thinking was right: I was a wuss. I continued to sit even with the revelation. It might have had something to do with the ribs, but that was just pain. Being hurt is way different from being a wuss. I've been hurt a lot, so this shouldn't be a problem.

In the revelation were also questions: What am I truly afraid of? What strikes the fear of God through my bones? Is it stacking end over end on my surfboard? Is it suffocation?

I don't think so.

I know that when I was drowning, twice, it wasn't horrific. I didn't feel panic, the white-knuckle fear that I would have expected.

What I feared, and still do, is the loss of connection. It's a question of the *who*. Not the wipeout. I fear relying on my faith, putting my trust in hope, and then having love ripped away. I fear raising my son only to rush him to the ER with an all-encompassing and life-ending bacterial infection. I fear choosing to get Chinese food when I should have just cooked some leftovers.

Once upon a time there was a boy who wanted to be a fighter pilot. There was a boy in his room acting like a surgeon, saving Bugs's life . . . every time. But all of that was just that: a dream. It was a vision of what I wanted, and what I thought I could be. It was a vision of this notion of winning and losing. But that was a romantic view of life. It is not the real world, real life. And it didn't get to the heart of my fear.

I worry about so many things, but I'm starting to realize they are the wrong things. It isn't like a switch that happens all at once. That's too contrived. I have to remind myself of these thoughts every day.

Just last night I had a conversation with my wife. I told her I had to finish *Fragile*.

We weren't connecting on the gravity of the task at hand. She made a comment that she might need help with the kids. She wasn't sure I could have a "day off" for my release and "fun."

There is no part of this that is "fun." Just so you know. I don't like writing. Donald Miller once said that he hated to write but loved to have written. I'm not even sure that is the case. I'm not sure how anyone will take this book. I might end up just feeling embarrassed. Hell, when I took the MCAT, the medical college admission test, I smoked it . . . except for the writing sample. On that section I scored abysmally, so maybe I don't even know what I'm doing here sitting and writing at this computer.

Fragile has been a chore. A literal tear-jerking chore. Sometimes I've written with coffee, listening to uplifting music. Other times, I've written with whiskey, NF playing in the background. But I've always tried to be honest.

What I mean is that I'm trying to be honest with myself. You get to be the voyeur this time, like me at the funeral.

Anyone who takes care of patients, has watched a love one suffer or die, or has put someone else in front of themselves may have some level of connection and understanding. And that's what I'm hoping for.

I needed to struggle through this to figure out my truth. And as I said before, there is no answer.

I wasn't even asking myself the right question. I would sit and ponder the *why*. But "Why?" is the wrong question. I should be focused on *who*.

And with all that, the conclusion leads to this: Worrying is a straight-up waste of time. Life is beyond control. Life is fragile. And because it is fragile it is unbelievably good.

Sitting on this beach, staring at the surf from the safety of the sand, is just like my life. I can live my life the way I surf. It's my choice. I can either sit on the edge of the swell, hang out on the shore, or man up and grab my board.

I might be just a fleck on the face of the universe, only one me in an infinite number of me's, but I'm not going to be *that* guy, *that* me. I'm not going to be the me who doesn't try. Who's afraid to try. I don't want to fear faith, or hope, or ultimately love. Because if I give in to that, then really, I have nothing. I might as well take the bailout now.

I want to be the me who all the other me's want to jump through the wormhole to be. I want to be the me who is going to wring out every last ounce of experience from this life. The one right here, right now, who wrote this book, these very words, not a better book.

Hell yeah, I'm afraid. But being afraid, that's good. Being afraid means I'm doing it right. It means I love my wife and kids so much that I can't imagine my world existing without them. It means I am proud of the work I've done to get to where I am. It means I value my life. It means I'm living. It means I'm asking the right question.

This world is scary. Just like paddling out into a big wave, it holds the potential for badness, things that I don't even want to think about. But, man, a good ride, that's exhilarating. Catching a wave feels incredible. It feels so good not just because of the rush of water underneath you, but because of all the other alternatives and possibilities. Being sucked out the back, slammed into the sand, flipped every which way, killed—as Jesse said—"dead, dead." That is the reason the ride is so gratifying.

I thought that somehow I could control everything. I was so wrong. Control is a myth. And being the master of the universe, it isn't even worth it. Because I don't know what I need, or even what I want.

For so much of my life I had been sitting on the sidelines. Just like I was now, on the beach, watching the others out in the swell. I was missing the point. Really, I was sitting on the edge of the vulnerability of letting people in, letting them get to the real me. I had to keep everything at arm's length just to be safe, just to function. I didn't truly want to love, all in, because that was dangerous.

I realized that I feared death. But in doing so, I was truly afraid to live. The living risked loss. I was afraid to try. To ride.

I made a choice, sitting on the beach, fighting the sense of being a wuss, of fearing the unknown. I changed my mind. No more. I was going all in. Because all this metaphorical crap is killing me. I needed to loosen my grip. Like, really loosen my grip.

This isn't easy. I had fooled myself that I would learn about life and death as a doctor without every coming face-to-face with death, suffering, loss. It sounds ridiculous when I put it that way, but it just might be true. I know now that, as embarrassing as my naiveté sounds, I needed to go into that rabbit hole, the hurt cave with no flashlight. I needed to sit in the hallway of a hospital, late at night, fluorescent lights blazing, head in my hands, pushing back the tears. I thought I was weak, that I wasn't cut out for medicine, that I wasn't good enough for this, my patients and their families. But that is exactly the place I needed to be.

There is no way I can feel love, happiness, and joy if I haven't felt the opposite. One is irrelevant without the other. The backdrop is what lets me feel the emotion, and only when emotions or feelings are placed in context, the context of a whole life, can I really start to be a fullhearted and content me.

On the beach, I remembered my envy of Steve and Joss's love, the sense of loss with Samuel, the smell of the helicopter fuel. I remembered all the people who had no choice but to hang on and ride. Life is truly crazy and unknown. Like any good story there needs to be adventure, intrigue, peril, and exhilaration. Anything less is boring.

That's why I don't want the infinity me. Sitting outside the break is pointless. I had protected myself from the very things that were most important. I needed to let Stephanie in, completely. I needed to feel completely vulnerable because she was so valuable. I can't live without her. And because she knows I'm weakened without her, I gain tremendous strength when she lays her hand on my insomniac head or holds my hand tightly when bagpipes start to play.

Life is always moving forward, like a wave. It only becomes completely available when I'm all in. I'm scared, and the fear opens the love. It enhances the emotion, all of it. Stephanie and my kids, my family, and all they bring fill my life to the complete spectrum.

This book is heavy. I know it is for me. But I want you to leave with something. More than just a feeling of death and dying or lack of control. I want you to feel things about your own life. I want you to take a moment, lie back, the way I did, and think about your own world. What do you fear? Think about the *who*.

I started this process as someone filled with doubt. I was someone who was swearing at God. But that vulnerability is what allowed the change; it allowed me to grow. Life isn't perfect. There isn't a magic formula for me because I toiled away at this book. But what I've come to realize is that it is OK.

I steadied myself on the shore, stood up, and spit into the sand. That was my way of being defiant, of convincing my mind that I'm tough. I got back into the water. Lying down on my board was painful, but really, it was nothing. Pain never ended anyone. I paddled out to the edge of the break. Breathing deep, taking in the sound of the seagulls and surf, I looked back for the next set. My body was telling me not to do it. But that didn't matter. I knew who I was. I wasn't going to quit. I was going to surf, to try to ride as if my life depended on it. Because as far as I could tell, when I compare the guy I was before I thought about all this to the guy I am now, my life did depend on it. Waves were coming, as sure as the moon circles the Earth. I didn't know if I'd ride or bulldozer my face into the sand, but that's life. As I bobbed up and down, anxiously waiting on the set, I knew one thing. I was going to paddle like a motherfucker.

EPILOGUE

WORK

"The Guardian Suite" Trevor Rabin

I t was 6:00 a.m. I hit the alarm on the phone. Why does that thing sound so chipper? It was cold. I think the thermostat was set to sixty-five. The temp outside was probably fifteen. I looked out the window. It even *looked* cold. Things were crisp, and white covered the ground. My truck was shrouded in pure, glistening snow. I wish I had an automatic start, like the new Dodge Ram my buddy just bought.

I showered and put on a fresh set of scrubs. Downstairs was quiet. The kids and my wife were still asleep. I grabbed a cup of coffee. In fact, counter to my normal prep, I had programmed the coffee machine the night before.

I stood by the kitchen window and looked out. It was beautiful. I would have never dreamed of anything so magnificent. Colorado is spectacular. My life is good. Not because I don't have bad days. Not because people don't die. Just the opposite.

I was mentally preparing for work. Later today, I could find myself standing in the docs' lounge trying to drown out *SportsCenter*—again dealing with the aftermath of Room 11. I could also find myself moved by a simple moment, unbelievably in love with my kids and my wife.

I know that I'm living because I was embracing all possibilities. I was on the journey, accepting whatever path unfolded. There was no way to win or lose. All I could do was loosen my grip and swing. Strikeout or home run. I was open to the spectrum. All of it. And it felt good.

Medicine is my home. It brings me to people at their core—true emotion, raw moments. The kind of experiences that make me live in the now. They make me enjoy the rainbow, actually see the rainbow. My wife's smile, with her nose crinkled so I know it's real. My son's band concert and his quirky music teacher. A jiujitsu tournament, a car ride, the dogs jumping into a lake. Amazing things. Brilliant moments that make me, in that moment, lose all interest in wormholes, other dimensions, or alternative me's.

I remind myself daily that this is exactly where I want to be. Feeling it all. The opposite of the zebra. Real life, happening in real time, big forward, small back. I need to let life happen. Surf the wave. All I need to do is get out of my own way, loosen my grip. Paddle. Ride.

As I looked out the window in my kitchen, I thought of a thousand things I would rather be doing today. I didn't want to go to work. But that didn't matter. This was my choice. It was my job. My innocence was lost.

Thankfully.

Because it forced me to have more faith. It led to my hope, in this life, here and now, even when things seem messed up. And with my faith and hope, I was able to find true love, for my wife and my family. I truly was able to discover the things I hold most dear.

And so I put on my black down jacket, along with my 49ers ski hat. Grabbing the scraper, I headed outside into the cold and white. I climbed in the truck and blew a crisp cloud out of my mouth. I put it in drive. The tires gripped as the wheels started to rotate. Another day of life and death in the ER—beauty in chaos, grace in tragedy, and the hope that lives in between.

ABOUT THE AUTHOR

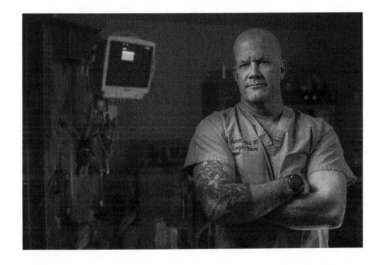

Shannon Sovndal, MD, produces the *Match on a Fire: Medicine and More* podcast and is the founder of 3Hundred Training Group. He is a board-certified doctor in both emergency medicine and emergency medical services (EMS). Dr. Sovndal attended medical school at Columbia University, where he earned the prestigious Arnold P. Gold Foundation Humanism in Medicine Award, and he completed residency in emergency medicine at Stanford University. He is a fellow of the American College of Emergency Physicians and has worked extensively in prehospital medicine, the fire service, and tactical medicine. He is currently the medical director for numerous air and ground EMS agencies and works with the Denver FBI Tactical Team. He has served on the board of directors for the Association of Air Medical Services and is the medical director for the Rocky Mountain Tactical Team Association. Dr. Sovndal has also worked at the Clinical Translational Research Center at the University of Colorado as a staff physician and was the team physician for the Garmin Professional Cycling Team, Slipstream Sports. He is the author of *Cycling Anatomy* and *Fitness Cycling.* He lives in Boulder, Colorado, with his family.

Made in the USA
Middletown, DE
19 August 2020